The Complete Diabetic Diet Cookbook for Beginners

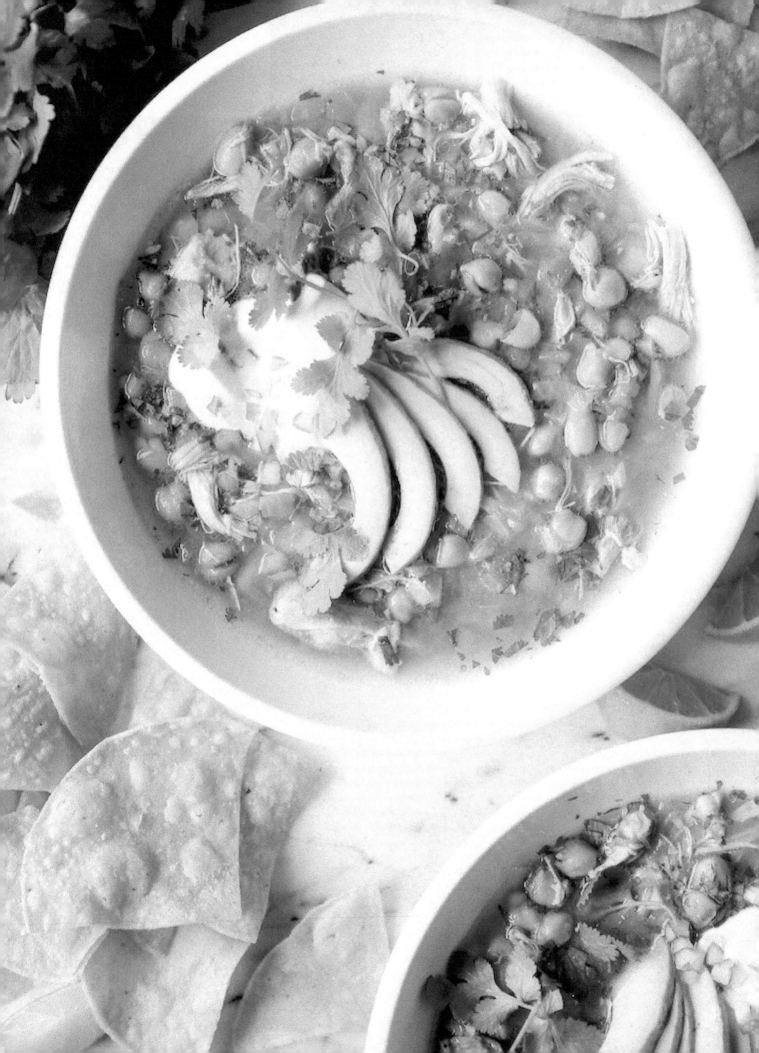

THE COMPLETE
DIABETIC DIET
COOKBOOK FOR BEGINNERS

600 | Easy and Healthy Diabetic Recipes for the Newly Diagnosed to Manage Prediabetes and Type 2 Diabetes

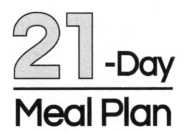

21-Day
Meal Plan

MELISSA S. STENNIS

CONTENT

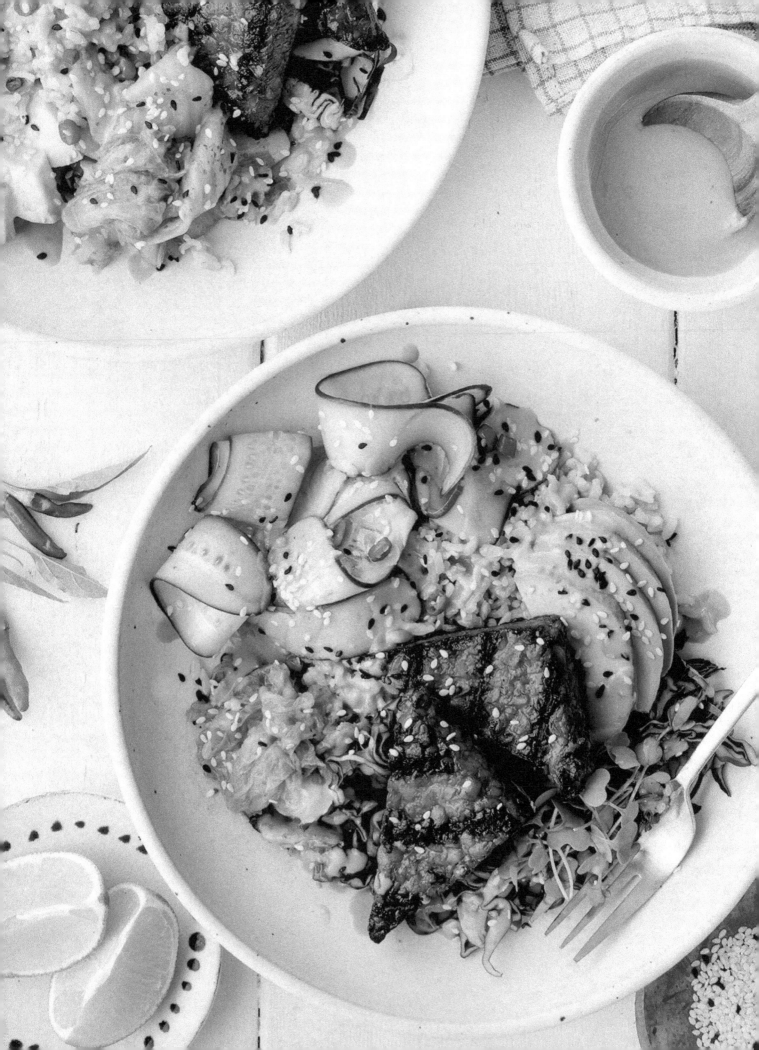

Introduction

Most of us know of someone in our circle of family or friends who lives with either type 1 or type 2 diabetes. Maybe we don't know who they are? And maybe that's because they don't talk to us about it? If we know who it is, maybe it's because we feel reluctant to ask them too many questions about their condition, because we are afraid to seem impolite. But, if we want to understand their condition, we really should ask them some questions. We should all become much more informed about the condition generally, so that we can help our friends and family members who have diabetes, to manage their health-care regime and stay well. Besides, we should all take be taking good care of our own general health, through sensible diet and regular exercise, to help prevent the onset of type 2 diabetes, and other related health conditions, as we get older. It's just common sense.

Statistics are often seen as a boring subject, and people don't want to pay too much attention to them, but these recent figures from the World Health Organization are some that we should all look at closely. You might actually find them a little alarming.

Studies in 2014 showed that the number of people who have diabetes rose from 108 million in 1980 to 422 million in 2014. By 2014, more than 8.5% of adults aged 18 years and older had diabetes across the globe. That's one person in every eight! By the year 2016, diabetes was the direct cause of 1.6 million deaths worldwide. Even more alarmingly, the global prevalence of diabetes among adults over 18 years of age rose from 4.7% in 1980 to 8.5% in 2014. Almost double the numbers! Things have not improved: between 2000 and 2016, there was a 5% increase in premature mortality from diabetes. And it is not just the "Developing" countries that swell the figures. In both high-income and low-income countries around the world, the premature mortality rate, directly due to diabetes, increased significantly in the six years between 2010 and 2016. These are figures that we absolutely cannot afford to ignore, as governments, or as individuals.

This easy-to-follow, recipe-packed cookbook will help you to guide yourself towards a lifestyle of healthier eating. If you are not diabetic, the recipes are simply a healthy and delicious way to take care of your blood sugar-levels and carb. Intake and prevent obesity. If you are diabetic, these recipes will enable you to live your life to the fullest, and to really enjoy preparing tasty meals that are fun to cook. But before you begin to try out the recipes on your family and friends, you really do need to understand what the condition is all about. We will answer some simple questions for you to help get you started: What are the differences between types 1 and 2 diabetes? Why are lifestyle choices and changes, such as quitting smoking, not drinking too much alcohol too frequently, eating sensibly, and taking regular exercise so important?

Chapter 1 Understanding Type 2 Diabetes

The condition that is commonly known as diabetes occurs when your pancreas does not produce enough insulin — this is a hormone that regulates the movement of sugar into your cells — and your cells react negatively, and respond poorly to insulin, so they take in less sugar.

What is Insulin? How Does It Work?

Insulin is a hormone that comes from the gland that is situated behind and below your stomach (it's called the pancreas). Insulin regulates how your body uses sugar in the following ways:

- Sugar in the bloodstream triggers the pancreas to secrete insulin.
- Insulin circulates in the bloodstream, enabling sugar to enter your cells.
- The amount of sugar in your bloodstream drops.
- In response to this drop, the pancreas releases less insulin.

It's pretty straightforward how it works, but keeping it regulated when you have type 2 diabetes is critical.

Type 2 diabetes is the most common form of diabetes. It is an impairment in the way that your body regulates and uses sugar as a fuel. This condition results in too much sugar circulating around your bloodstream. Eventually, these high blood sugar levels can lead to disorders of the circulatory, nervous and immune systems. In type 2 diabetes, there are, primarily, two problems. These are short-term problems, and long-term problems. That is to say, symptoms, and complications. These are listed to help you to see the differences.

There is no cure for type 2 diabetes. Losing weight, eating well, and exercising can help manage the condition. If diet and exercise aren't effective, you may also need medication or insulin therapy. Please note: No-one should ever undertake any radical diet or lifestyle changes without first consulting a medical doctor. Risk factors for type 2 diabetes include some lifestyle choices that can be reduced or removed entirely when I am talking about "risk factors and lifestyle choices" in this context, I am referring directly to obesity and lack of exercise.

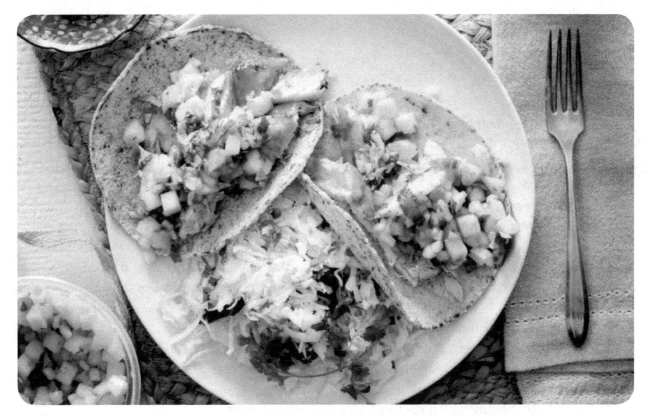

Significant risk factors include:

- Ageing/growing older
- Excess weight, particularly around the waist
- Family history
- Certain ethnicities
- Physical inactivity
- Poor diet

Prevalence: Type 2 diabetes accounts for approximately 90 to 95 percent of all diagnosed cases of diabetes in adults. Research suggests that 1 out of 3 adults has prediabetes. More than one in every 10 adults who are 20 years or older has diabetes. For seniors (65 years and older), that figure rises to more than one in four.

Signs and symptoms of type 2 diabetes develop slowly. In fact, you can be living with type 2 diabetes for years and not even know it! If signs and symptoms are present, they may include some of the following:

- Increased thirst
- Frequent urination
- Increased hunger
- Unintended weight loss
- Fatigue
- Blurred vision
- Slow-healing sores
- Frequent infections
- Numbness or tingling in the hands or feet
- Areas of darkened skin, usually in the armpits and neck

Type 2 diabetes affects your major organs: your heart, blood vessels, nerves, eyes and kidneys. In addition to these effects, factors that increase the risk of diabetes are also risk factors for other very serious, chronic diseases. So, managing diabetes and controlling your blood sugar levels can lower your risk for complications or coexisting conditions as you get older.

Potential complications of diabetes:

- **Heart and blood vessel disease.** Diabetes is associated with an increased risk of heart disease, stroke, high blood pressure and narrowing of the blood vessels and arteries (atherosclerosis).
- **Nerve damage in limbs.** Consistently high blood sugar levels over time can damage or destroy nerves, resulting in tingling, numbness, burning, pain or eventual loss of feeling that usually begins at the tips of the toes or fingers and gradually spreads upward. This puts you at risk of injuring yourself without knowing about it until you are badly hurt.
- **Other nerve damage.** Damage to nerves of the heart can contribute to irregular heart rhythms. Nerve damage in the digestive system can cause problems with nausea, vomiting, diarrhea or constipation. For men, nerve damage may cause erectile dysfunction.
- **Kidney disease.** Diabetes may lead to chronic kidney disease or irreversible end-stage kidney disease, which may require dialysis or a kidney transplant.
- **Eye damage.** Diabetes increases the risk of serious eye diseases, such as cataracts and glaucoma, and may damage the blood vessels of the retina, potentially leading to blindness.
- **Skin conditions** - including bacterial and fungal infections.
- **Slow healing** - untreated cuts and blisters can become serious infections, which may heal poorly. Severe damage to limbs might even require amputation.
- **Hearing impairment** - hearing problems are more common in people with diabetes.
- **Sleep apnoea** - Obstructive Sleep Apnoea is common in people with type 2 diabetes. Obesity may be the main contributing factor to both conditions. This condition is seriously detrimental to overall quality of life, and can cause premature death though heart failure, due to lack of oxygen in the blood.
- **Dementia** - the risk of Alzheimer's disease and other disorders that cause dementia are significantly increased. Poor control of blood sugar levels is linked to a more rapid decline in overall memory, and other critical thinking skills.

What is the Difference between Type 1 Diabetes and Type 2 Diabetes?

The two most common forms of diabetes are type 1 and type 2. Both involve problems with insulin, but the causes of type 1 and type 2 diabetes are different.

People with type 1 diabetes don't produce insulin and they need to rely on insulin injections in order to survive. Type 1 is an autoimmune condition, in which your immune system targets the insulin-producing cells in your pancreas. It has a genetic component. However, not all identical twins get type 1 diabetes, so other factors may play a role in which people are most susceptible to the condition.

People with type 2 diabetes do produce insulin, but they are unable to use their own insulin effectively, either because they don't make enough or because their cells are resistant to the insulin that they do make. People with type 2 can use a combination of diet, exercise, oral medication, and insulin or other injectable drugs to control their blood sugar.

What is a Healthy Diet for Someone with Diabetes?

When you have type 1 diabetes, you can eat pretty much the same diet as anyone else, provided it is a healthy diet that is low in unhealthy fats. There are some rules, that you should follow though:

Meal timing is very important for people. Your meals must match insulin doses. Eating meals with a low glycaemic index makes meal timing easier. Low glycaemic loads raise your blood sugar slowly and steadily, which leaves plenty of time for your body (or the injected insulin dose you take) to respond. Skipping a meal or eating late puts you at risk for low blood sugar (hypoglycaemia).

Foods you should eat if you are type 1 include complex carbohydrates such as these:

- Brown rice
- Whole wheat
- Quinoa
- Oatmeal
- Fruits
- Vegetables
- Beans and Lentils

Foods that you should avoid if you are type 1 include the following:

- Sodas (both diet and regular)
- Simple carbohydrates - processed/refined sugars, like white bread, pastries, chips, cookies, pasta
- Trans fats (anything with the word hydrogenated on the label) and high-fat animal products. Fats don't have much of a direct effect on blood sugar, but they can be useful in slowing the absorption of carbohydrates.

When you have type 2 diabetes, you should follow a meal plan that includes complex carbohydrates such as those listed above. Foods to avoid include the same simple carbohydrates - such as sugar, pasta, white bread, flour, cookies, and pastries, etc. So, it's similar to how you should eat if you have type 1. A high protein diet provides steady energy with little effect on blood sugar, and can help with sugar cravings and feeling full after eating. Protein-packed foods to eat include beans, legumes, eggs, seafood, dairy, peas, tofu, and lean meats and poultry. All these are easy to cook, easy to access foods. And, if you want to give your diet a boost, there are five diabetes "superfoods" that you can eat, which are very beneficial to the cardio-vascular system, digestion, and general health. These include chia seeds, wild salmon, white balsamic vinegar, cinnamon, and lentils.

As with any healthy-eating program, a healthy diabetes meal plan should include plenty of vegetables, and limit amounts of processed sugars and red meat. For people with type 2 diabetes, dietitians often recommend a vegetarian or vegan diet. If you really want to eat meat, the Paleo Diet, and the Mediterranean Diet are also recommended.

How Much Should I Eat Per Day?

First of all, how many calories you are taking in depends on whether or not you are taking insulin with your meals (type 1.) If you take mealtime insulin, you need to count carbs to match your insulin dose to the amount of carbs in your foods and drinks. You may also take additional insulin if your blood sugar is higher than your target when eating. So, this will affect amounts of insulin that you self-administer on a daily basis.

If you are Type 2, then you are not taking insulin with your meals, so life is a little less complicated. But you still have to count the carbs if you want to maintain your blood sugar levels. Everyone, whether they have type 1 or type 2 diabetes or not, should be eating a balanced, nutritious diet that is appropriate for their age and their activity levels. Staying hydrated is critical too. Drinking lots of water is an important part of maintaining good general health.

Nutrition and Diabetes

Nutrition is not simply about how much you eat, it's also about what you eat. And, as we have touched on already, if you have diabetes, it's also about when you eat. It is probable, if you have type 2 diabetes, that you are overweight. So, losing a few of those excess kilos is absolutely essential. Meal planning is, therefore, very important, because random "grazing" is not a good way to control what we eat. Becoming generally more active, and then making big changes to what you eat and drink can seem very challenging at first. Especially if your bad habits are ingrained. You may find it easier to start by making some small changes, and it won't hurt to get some help and support from your family, friends, and health care team. Eating well and being physically active most days of the week can help you with the essentials of well-being and managing your condition:

- Keeping your blood glucose level, blood pressure, and cholesterol in your target ranges
- Losing weight or maintaining a healthy weight
- Preventing or delaying diabetes problems
- Feeling good and having more energy

You need to eat a variety of healthy foods, from all the food groups, in the exact amounts that your diabetic meal plan outlines.

The food groups are:

Vegetables
- Non-starchy vegetables include broccoli, carrots, greens, peppers, and tomatoes
- Starchy vegetables include potatoes, corn, and green peas

Fruits (oranges, melon, berries, apples, bananas, and grapes etc)

Grains (at least half of your grains for the day should be whole grains)
- wheat, rice, oats, cornmeal, barley, and quinoa
- bread, pasta, cereal, and tortillas

Protein
- Lean meat
- Chicken or turkey without the skin
- Fish
- Eggs
- Nuts and peanuts
- Dried beans and certain peas, such as chickpeas and split peas
- Meat substitutes, such as tofu

Dairy (non-fat or low fat preferably)
- Milk or lactose-free milk if you are lactose intolerant
- Yogurt
- Cheese

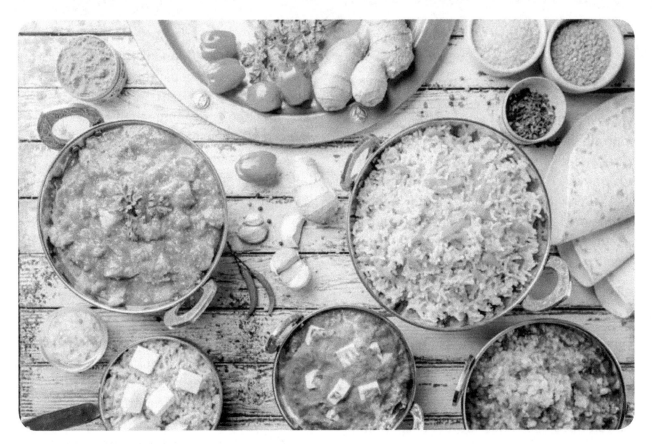

Exercise and Diabetes

Exercise is an important part of everyone's healthy life, and it is critical to your diabetes treatment plan. To avoid potential problems, make sure that you check your blood sugar before, during, and after you exercise. This will show you how your body responds to exercise, and this can help you to prevent potentially dangerous blood sugar fluctuations. If you are taking insulin or other medications that can cause low blood sugar (hypoglycaemia), it is vital that you test your blood sugar 15 to 30 minutes before you start exercising. If you don't take medications for your diabetes or you don't use medications commonly linked to low blood sugar levels, you probably won't need to take any special precautions prior to exercising. But it is a good habit to get into anyway. If you are in any doubt, check with your doctor.

Before you get started on your exercise program, ask your doctor how the activities that you're contemplating might affect your blood sugar. The doctor can also suggest the optimum time to exercise, and he can explain the potential impact of medications on your blood sugar as you become more active.

Health experts recommend that everyone, irrespective of whether they are diabetic or not, undertakes at least 150 minutes per week of moderately intense physical activities such as:

- Fast walking
- Lap swimming
- Bicycling

But once you are feeling an improvement in your overall energy levels, and your fitness and stamina has built up, you can take your exercise routine to higher levels. Always remember to check those blood sugar levels and consult your doctor before you make any significant changes.

Tips and Tricks

We have included a couple of easy things that you can do on a day-to-day basis that will make the planning and preparation of your meals so much easier. It's always good to be aware of what you are putting into your body anyway, but it's super-important when you have diabetes. So, understanding what food is made up of is important. You might be surprised by what is in some of those "healthy" foods that you regularly eat!

How to read a label

Understanding the Nutrition Facts labels on pre-prepared and processed food items will help you to make much healthier choices. Labels usually break down the percentages of calories, carbs, fats, fibres, proteins, and vitamins per serving. This makes it easier for you to compare the nutritional content and value of similar products. Look at different brands of the same foods—nutrition information can differ a lot. One brand of tomato sauce may have more calories and sugar than another brand, for the same serving size. Next time you go shopping, look at the labels of the most common items in your cupboards and refrigerator, and compare them with other brands of the same. You can photograph the labels with your smartphone for an accurate comparison with items in the store as you shop.

Counting Carbohydrates

Carb counting simply involves counting the number of grams of carbohydrate that are in a meal and then matching that to your dose of insulin. If you take mealtime insulin, first account for each carbohydrate gram you eat, and dose your mealtime insulin based on that count. It's what's known as an insulin-to-carb ratio, and it calculates how much insulin you should take to manage your blood sugars after eating. This form of carb counting is recommended for people who are on intensive insulin therapy. If you don't need to take insulin, you can do a more basic version of carb counting based on "carbohydrate choices." Put simply, this is where one "choice" contains about 15 grams of carbohydrate. Or, you could try using the Diabetes Plate Method by limiting whole grains, starchy vegetables, fruits or dairy to a quarter of your plate.

Try Creating a 21-Day Diabetic Meal Plan

While some meal plans cater specifically to exercise, most cater more to dietary choices, such as restricting calories, fitting specific macro and micronutrient profiles, avoiding inflammatory foods, and so on. In the case of a diabetic meal plan, carbohydrate counting and glycaemic levels or different foods are important.

Beyond just exercise routines and dietary guidelines, this meal plan offers the additional support of the recipes in this cookbook.

There are many meal plans these days, with accompanying programs that cater to just about any dietary preference or need that you can think of.

These are just a few of the different types of weight loss programs available:
• Vegetarian
• Vegan
• Keto
• Paleo
• Diabetes support
• Gluten free

Even if you find it hard to follow a program that is tailored to your specific needs, this 21-day meal plan will really help you to understand what you need to do to maintain good diabetic health.

So, eat well, and stay healthy!

21-Day Meal Plan

DAYS	BREAKFAST	LUNCH	DINNER	SNACK/ DESSERT
1	Berry-Coconut Smoothie Bowl [12]	Cucumber Tomato Avocado Salad [42]	One-Pot Roast Chicken Dinner [86]	Baked Parmesan Crisps [47]
2	Avocado Goat Cheese Toast [13]	Zoodles with Beet and Walnut Pesto [59]	Honey Ginger Glazed Salmon with Broccoli [119]	Grilled Peach and Coconut Yogurt Bowls [136]
3	Cinnamon Walnut Granola [14]	Saffron Chicken [78]	Beef Curry [102]	No-Bake Carrot Cake Bites [132]
4	Chocolate Zucchini Muffins [20]	Bunless Sloppy Joes [103]	Chicken Cacciatore [89]	Creamy Strawberry Crepes [135]
5	Carrot Oat Pancakes [22]	Blackberry Goat Cheese Salad [49]	Whole Veggie-Stuffed Trout [118]	Buffalo Chicken Celery Sticks [47]
6	Breakfast Pita with Egg and Bacon [19]	Lemon Pepper Salmon [119]	Turkey and Quinoa Caprese Casserole [83]	Maple Oatmeal Cookies [132]
7	Sausage and Pepper Breakfast Burrito [25]	Teriyaki Meatballs [76]	Halibut Roasted with Green Beans [124]	Zucchini Hummus Dip with Red Peppers [47]
8	Canadian Bacon and Egg Muffin Cups [16]	Squash and Barley Salad [51]	Savory Rubbed Roast Chicken [77]	Banana Pudding [141]
9	Tropical Steel Cut Oats [20]	Ceviche [126]	Lamb Burgers with Mushrooms and Cheese [101]	Cocoa Coated Almonds [43]
10	Cranberry Almond Grits [23]	Brussels Sprouts Wild Rice Bowl [60]	Blackened Tilapia with Mango Salsa [127]	Spiced Orange Rice Pudding [133]

11	Berry Almond Smoothie [15]	Mustard Glazed Pork Chops [99]	Shredded Buffalo Chicken [87]	Apple Crunch [138]
12	Blueberry Coconut Breakfast Cookies [14]	Quinoa, Salmon, and Avocado Salad [54]	Beef and Butternut Squash Stew [107]	Garlic Kale Chips [47]
13	Coconut Pancakes [18]	Chicken and Onion Grilled Cheese [79]	Lemon Butter Cod with Asparagus [125]	Chai Pear-Fig Compote [138]
14	Breakfast Tacos [26]	Cajun Shrimp and Quinoa Casserole [128]	Braised Chicken with Grape-Apple Slaw [91]	Peanut Butter Protein Bites [45]
15	Sausage, Sweet Potato, and Kale Hash [22]	Thai Shrimp Soup [28]	Roasted Pork Loin [100]	Goat Cheese-Stuffed Pears [135]
16	Maple Sausage Frittata [16]	Ratatouille [63]	Teriyaki Chicken and Broccoli [93]	Chipotle Black Bean Brownies [141]
17	Ham and Cheese English Muffin Melt [16]	Ground Turkey Taco Skillet [83]	Shrimp with Tomatoes and Feta [122]	Ice Cream with Strawberry Rhubarb Sauce [133]
18	Pumpkin Walnut Smoothie Bowl [17]	Lime Chicken Tortilla Soup [32]	Sunday Pot Roast [108]	Cinnamon Toasted Pumpkin Seeds [43]
19	Avocado Toast with Tomato and Cheese [18]	Fish Tacos [120]	Chicken and Roasted Vegetable Wraps [86]	Guacamole with Jicama [47]
20	Broccoli and Mushroom Frittata [23]	Baked Tofu and Mixed Vegetable Bowl [67]	Pork and Apple Skillet [104]	Broiled Pineapple [137]
21	Heart-Healthy Yogurt Parfaits [17]	Open-Faced Philly Cheesesteak Sandwiches [100]	Salmon Florentine [124]	Buckwheat Crêpes with Fruit and Yogurt [140]

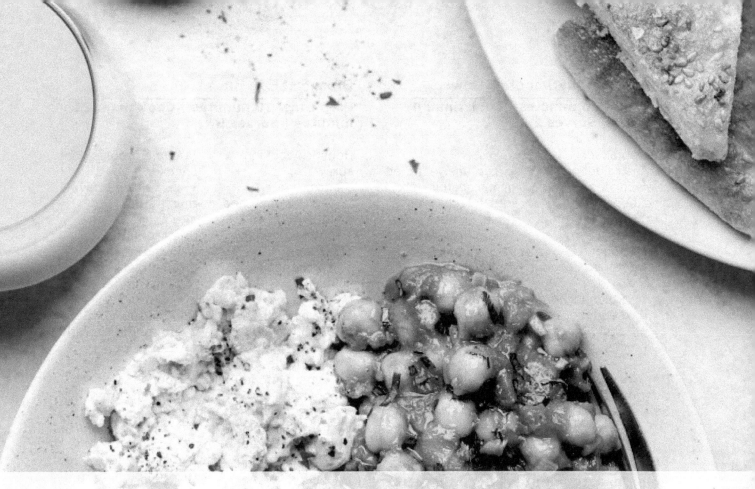

Chapter 2 Breakfast

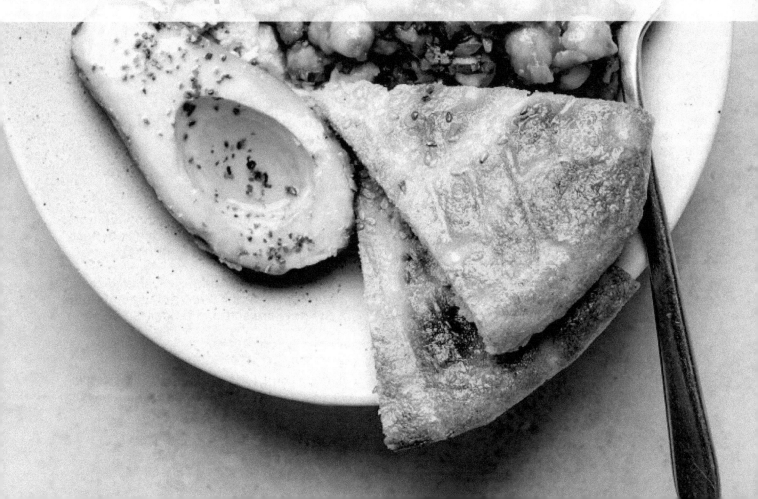

Berry-Coconut Smoothie Bowl

Prep time: 5 minutes | Cook time: 0 minutes | Serves 2

½ cup mixed berries (blueberries, strawberries, blackberries)
1 tablespoon ground flaxseed
2 tablespoons unsweetened coconut
flakes
½ cup unsweetened plain coconut milk
½ cup leafy greens (kale, spinach)
¼ cup unsweetened vanilla nonfat yogurt
½ cup ice

1. In a blender jar, combine the berries, flaxseed, coconut flakes, coconut milk, greens, yogurt, and ice.
2. Process until smooth. Serve.

Per Serving
calories: 180 | fat: 15g | protein: 8g | carbs: 8g | sugars: 3g | fiber: 4g | sodium: 24mg

Spinach Artichoke Egg Casserole

Prep time: 10 minutes | Cook time: 35 minutes | Serves 8

Nonstick cooking spray
1 (10-ounce / 283-g) package frozen spinach, thawed and drained
1 (14-ounce / 397-g) can artichoke hearts, drained
¼ cup finely chopped red bell pepper
2 garlic cloves, minced
8 eggs, lightly beaten
¼ cup unsweetened plain almond milk
½ teaspoon salt
½ teaspoon freshly ground black pepper
½ cup crumbled goat cheese

1. Preheat the oven to 375ºF (190ºC). Spray an 8-by-8-inch baking dish with nonstick cooking spray.
2. In a large mixing bowl, combine the spinach, artichoke hearts, bell pepper, garlic, eggs, almond milk, salt, and pepper. Stir well to combine.
3. Transfer the mixture to the baking dish. Sprinkle with the goat cheese.
4. Bake for 35 minutes until the eggs are set. Serve warm.

Per Serving
calories: 105 | fat: 5g | protein: 9g | carbs: 6g | sugars: 1g | fiber: 2g | sodium: 488mg

Breakfast Egg Bites

Prep time: 10 minutes | Cook time: 25 minutes | Serves 8

Nonstick cooking spray
6 eggs, beaten
¼ cup unsweetened plain almond milk
1 red bell pepper, diced
1 cup chopped spinach
¼ cup crumbled goat cheese
½ cup sliced brown mushrooms
¼ cup sliced sun-dried tomatoes
Salt and freshly ground black pepper, to taste

1. Preheat the oven to 350ºF (180ºC). Spray 8 muffin cups of a 12-cup muffin tin with nonstick cooking spray. Set aside.
2. In a large mixing bowl, combine the eggs, almond milk, bell pepper, spinach, goat cheese, mushrooms, and tomatoes. Season with salt and pepper.
3. Fill the prepared muffin cups three-fourths full with the egg mixture. Bake for 20 to 25 minutes until the eggs are set. Let cool slightly and remove the egg bites from the muffin tin.
4. Serve warm, or store in an airtight container in the refrigerator for up to 5 days or in the freezer for up to 1 month.

Per Serving
calories: 68 | fat: 4g | protein: 6g | carbs: 3g | sugars: 2g | fiber: 1g | sodium: 126mg

Savory Corn Grits

Prep time: 5 minutes | Cook time: 7 minutes | Serves 4

2 cups water
1 cup fat-free milk
1 cup stone-ground corn grits

1. In a heavy-bottomed pot, bring the water and milk to a simmer over medium heat.
2. Gradually add the grits, stirring continuously.
3. Reduce the heat to low, cover, and cook, stirring often, for 5 to 7 minutes, or until the grits are soft and tender. Serve and enjoy.

Per Serving
calories: 166 | fat: 1g | protein: 6g | carbs: 34g | sugars: 3g | fiber: 1g | sodium: 32mg

Avocado Goat Cheese Toast

Prep time: 5 minutes | Cook time: 10 minutes | Serves 2

2 slices whole-wheat thin-sliced bread
½ avocado

2 tablespoons crumbled goat cheese
Salt, to taste

1. In a toaster or broiler, toast the bread until browned.
2. Remove the flesh from the avocado. In a medium bowl, use a fork to mash the avocado flesh. Spread it onto the toast.
3. Sprinkle with the goat cheese and season lightly with salt.
4. Add any toppings and serve.

Per Serving
calories: 137 | fat: 6g | protein: 5g | carbs: 18g | sugars: 0g | fiber: 5g | sodium: 195mg

Poached Eggs

Prep time: 5 minutes | Cook time: 5 minutes | Serves 4

Nonstick cooking spray

4 large eggs

1. Lightly spray 4 cups of a 7-count silicone egg bite mold with nonstick cooking spray. Crack each egg into a sprayed cup.
2. Pour 1 cup of water into the electric pressure cooker. Place the egg bite mold on the wire rack and carefully lower it into the pot.
3. Close and lock the lid of the pressure cooker. Set the valve to sealing.
4. Cook on high pressure for 5 minutes.
5. When the cooking is complete, hit Cancel and quick release the pressure.
6. Once the pin drops, unlock and remove the lid.
7. Run a small rubber spatula or spoon around each egg and carefully remove it from the mold. The white should be cooked, but the yolk should be runny.
8. Serve immediately.

Per Serving
calories: 78 | fat: 5g | protein: 6g | carbs: 1g | sugars: 0g | fiber: 0g | sodium: 62mg

Peanut Butter Power Oats

Prep time: 5 minutes | Cook time: 5 minutes | Serves 2

1½ cups unsweetened vanilla almond milk
¾ cup rolled oats
1 tablespoon chia seeds
2 tablespoons natural

peanut butter
2 tablespoons walnut pieces, divided (optional)
¼ cup fresh berries, divided (optional)

1. In a small saucepan, bring the almond milk, oats, and chia seeds to a simmer.
2. Cover and cook, stirring frequently, until all of the milk is absorbed, and the chia seeds have gelled.
3. Add the peanut butter and stir until creamy.
4. Divide the oatmeal between two bowls. Top each serving with half of the walnuts and/or berries (if using).

Per Serving
calories: 261 | fat: 14g | protein: 10g | carbs: 27g | sugars: 1g | fiber: 7g | sodium: 131mg

Homemade Turkey Breakfast Sausage

Prep time: 10 minutes | Cook time: 10 minutes | Serves 8

1 pound (454 g) lean ground turkey
½ teaspoon salt
½ teaspoon dried sage
½ teaspoon dried thyme

½ teaspoon freshly ground black pepper
¼ teaspoon ground fennel seeds
1 teaspoon extra-virgin olive oil

1. In a large mixing bowl, combine the ground turkey, salt, sage, thyme, pepper, and fennel. Mix well.
2. Shape the meat into 8 small, round patties.
3. Heat the olive oil in a skillet over medium-high heat. Cook the patties in the skillet for 3 to 4 minutes on each side until browned and cooked through.
4. Serve warm, or store in an airtight container in the refrigerator for up to 3 days or in the freezer for up to 1 month.

Per Serving
calories: 91 | fat: 5g | protein: 11g | carbs: 0g | sugars: 0g | fiber: 0g | sodium: 156mg

Yogurt Sundae

Prep time: 5 minutes | Cook time: 0 minutes | Serves 1

¾ cup plain nonfat Greek yogurt
¼ cup mixed berries (blueberries, strawberries, blackberries)
2 tablespoons

cashew, walnut, or almond pieces
1 tablespoon ground flaxseed
2 fresh mint leaves, shredded

1. Spoon the yogurt into a small bowl. Top with the berries, nuts, and flaxseed.
2. Garnish with the mint and serve.

Per Serving

calories: 238 | fat: 11g | protein: 21g | carbs: 16g | sugars: 9g | fiber: 4g | sodium: 64mg

Cinnamon Walnut Granola

Prep time: 10 minutes | Cook time: 30 minutes | Serves 16

4 cups rolled oats
1 cup walnut pieces
½ cup pepitas
¼ teaspoon salt
1 teaspoon ground cinnamon
1 teaspoon ground ginger

½ cup coconut oil, melted
½ cup unsweetened applesauce
1 teaspoon vanilla extract
½ cup dried cherries

1. Preheat the oven to 350°F (180°C). Line a baking sheet with parchment paper.
2. In a large bowl, toss the oats, walnuts, pepitas, salt, cinnamon, and ginger.
3. In a large measuring cup, combine the coconut oil, applesauce, and vanilla. Pour over the dry mixture and mix well.
4. Transfer the mixture to the prepared baking sheet. Cook for 30 minutes, stirring about halfway through. Remove from the oven and let the granola sit undisturbed until completely cool. Break the granola into pieces, and stir in the dried cherries.
5. Transfer to an airtight container, and store at room temperature for up to 2 weeks.

Per Serving

calories: 224 | fat: 15g | protein: 5g | carbs: 20g | sugars: 5g | fiber: 3g | sodium: 30mg

Tropical Greek Yogurt Bowl

Prep time: 5 minutes | Cook time: 0 minutes | Serves 2

1½ cups plain low-fat Greek yogurt
2 kiwis, peeled and sliced
2 tablespoons shredded unsweetened coconut

flakes
2 tablespoons halved walnuts
1 tablespoon chia seeds
2 teaspoons honey, divided (optional)

1. Divide the yogurt between two small bowls.
2. Top each serving of yogurt with half of the kiwi slices, coconut flakes, walnuts, chia seeds, and honey (if using).

Per Serving

calories: 260 | fat: 9g | protein: 21g | carbs: 23g | sugars: 14g | fiber: 6g | sodium: 83mg

Blueberry Coconut Breakfast Cookies

Prep time: 10 minutes | Cook time: 15 minutes | Serves 4

4 tablespoons unsalted butter, at room temperature
2 medium bananas
4 large eggs
½ cup unsweetened applesauce

1 teaspoon vanilla extract
⅔ cup coconut flour
¼ teaspoon salt
1 cup fresh or frozen blueberries

1. Preheat the oven to 375°F (190°C).
2. In a medium bowl, mash the butter and bananas together with a fork until combined. The bananas can be a little chunky.
3. Add the eggs, applesauce, and vanilla to the bananas and mix well.
4. Stir in the coconut flour and salt.
5. Gently fold in the blueberries.
6. Drop about 2 tablespoons of dough on a baking sheet for each cookie and flatten it a bit with the back of a spoon. Bake for about 13 minutes, or until firm to the touch.

Per Serving

calories: 305 | fat: 18g | protein: 8g | carbs: 28g | sugars: 15g | fiber: 7g | sodium: 222mg

6-Grain Porridge

Prep time: 5 minutes | Cook time: 20 minutes | Serves 7

½ cup steel cut oats
½ cup short-grain brown rice
½ cup millet
½ cup barley
⅓ cup wild rice
¼ cup corn grits or polenta (not instant)
3 tablespoons ground flaxseed

½ teaspoon salt
Ground cinnamon (optional)
Unsweetened almond milk (optional)
Berries (optional)
Sliced almonds or chopped walnuts (optional)

1. In the electric pressure cooker, combine the oats, brown rice, millet, barley, wild rice, grits, flaxseed, salt, and 8 cups of water.
2. Close and lock the lid of the pressure cooker. Set the valve to sealing.
3. Cook on high pressure for 20 minutes.
4. When the cooking is complete, hit Cancel and allow the pressure to release naturally for 15 minutes, then quick release any remaining pressure.
5. Once the pin drops, unlock and remove the lid. Stir.
6. Serve with any combination of cinnamon, almond milk, berries, and nuts (if using).

Per Serving (½ cup)
calories: 263 | fat: 3g | protein: 8g | carbs: 51g | sugars: 0g | fiber: 7g | sodium: 140mg

Berry Almond Smoothie

Prep time: 5 minutes | Cook time: 0 minutes | Serves 4

2 cups frozen berries of choice
1 cup plain low-fat Greek yogurt

1 cup unsweetened vanilla almond milk
½ cup natural almond butter

1. Put the berries, yogurt, almond milk, and almond butter into a blender and blend until smooth. If the smoothie is too thick, add more almond milk to thin.

Per Serving
calories: 277 | fat: 18g | protein: 13g | carbs: 19g | sugars: 11g | fiber: 6g | sodium: 140mg

Brussels Sprout Hash with Eggs

Prep time: 15 minutes | Cook time: 15 minutes | Serves 4

3 teaspoons extra-virgin olive oil, divided
1 pound (454 g) Brussels sprouts, sliced

2 garlic cloves, thinly sliced
¼ teaspoon salt
Juice of 1 lemon
4 eggs

1. In a large skillet, heat 1½ teaspoons of oil over medium heat. Add the Brussels sprouts and toss. Cook, stirring regularly, for 6 to 8 minutes until browned and softened. Add the garlic and continue to cook until fragrant, about 1 minute. Season with the salt and lemon juice. Transfer to a serving dish.
2. In the same pan, heat the remaining 1½ teaspoons of oil over medium-high heat. Crack the eggs into the pan. Fry for 2 to 4 minutes, flip, and continue cooking to desired doneness. Serve over the bed of hash.

Per Serving
calories: 158 | fat: 9g | protein: 10g | carbs: 12g | sugars: 4g | fiber: 4g | sodium: 234mg

Simple Grain-Free Biscuits

Prep time: 10 minutes | Cook time: 15 minutes | Serves 4

2 tablespoons unsalted butter
Pinch salt
¼ cup plain low-fat

Greek yogurt
1½ cups finely ground almond flour

1. Preheat the oven to 375ºF (190ºC).
2. In a medium bowl, microwave the butter just enough to soften, 15 to 20 seconds.
3. Add the salt and yogurt to the butter and mix well.
4. Add the almond flour and mix. The dough will be crumbly at first, so continue to stir and mash it with a fork until there are no lumps and the mixture comes together.
5. Drop ¼ cup of dough on a baking sheet for each biscuit. Using your clean hand, flatten each biscuit until it is 1 inch thick.
6. Bake for 13 to 15 minutes.

Per Serving
calories: 311 | fat: 28g | protein: 10g | carbs: 9g | sugars: 2g | fiber: 5g | sodium: 32mg

Maple Sausage Frittata

Prep time: 10 minutes | Cook time: 15 minutes | Serves 4

Avocado oil cooking spray
1 cup roughly chopped portobello mushrooms
1 medium green bell pepper, diced
1 medium red bell pepper, diced

8 large eggs
¾ cup half-and-half
¼ cup unsweetened almond milk
6 links maple-flavored chicken or turkey breakfast sausage, cut into ¼-inch pieces

1. Preheat the oven to 375ºF (190ºC).
2. Heat a large, oven-safe skillet over medium-low heat. When hot, coat the cooking surface with cooking spray.
3. Heat the mushrooms, green bell pepper, and red bell pepper in the skillet. Cook for 5 minutes.
4. Meanwhile, in a medium bowl, whisk the eggs, half-and-half, and almond milk.
5. Add the sausage to the skillet and cook for 2 minutes.
6. Pour the egg mixture into the skillet, then transfer the skillet from the stove to the oven, and bake for 15 minutes, or until the middle is firm and spongy.

Per Serving
calories: 280 | fat: 17g | protein: 21g | carbs: 10g | sugars: 7g | fiber: 2g | sodium: 446mg

Cinnamon Overnight Oats

Prep time: 5 minutes | Cook time: 0 minutes | Serves 1

$^1/_3$ cup unsweetened almond milk
$^1/_3$ cup rolled oats (use gluten-free if necessary)
¼ apple, cored and

finely chopped
2 tablespoons chopped walnuts
½ teaspoon cinnamon
Pinch sea salt

1. In a single-serving container or mason jar, combine all of the ingredients and mix well.
2. Cover and refrigerate overnight.

Per Serving
calories: 242 | fat: 12g | protein: 6g | carbs: 30g | sugars: 9g | fiber: 6g | sodium: 97mg

Ham and Cheese English Muffin Melt

Prep time: 10 minutes | Cook time: 5 minutes | Serves 2

1 whole-grain English muffin, split and toasted
2 teaspoons Dijon mustard
2 slices tomato

4 thin slices deli ham
½ cup shredded Cheddar cheese
2 large eggs, fried (optional)

1. Preheat the oven broiler on high.
2. Spread each toasted English muffin half with 1 teaspoon of mustard, and place them on a rimmed baking sheet, cut-side up.
3. Top each with a tomato slice and 2 slices of ham. Sprinkle each with half of the cheese.
4. Broil in the preheated oven until the cheese melts, 2 to 3 minutes.
5. Serve immediately, topped with a fried egg, if desired.

Per Serving
calories: 234 | fat: 13g | protein: 16g | carbs: 16g | sugars: 0g | fiber: 3g | sodium: 834mg

Canadian Bacon and Egg Muffin Cups

Prep time: 5 minutes | Cook time: 20 minutes | Serves 6

Cooking spray (for greasing)
6 large slices Canadian bacon
12 large eggs, beaten
1 teaspoon Dijon

mustard
½ teaspoon sea salt
Dash hot sauce
1 cup shredded Swiss cheese

1. Preheat the oven to 350ºF (180ºC). Spray 6 nonstick muffin cups with cooking spray.
2. Line each cup with 1 slice of Canadian bacon.
3. In a bowl, whisk together the eggs, mustard, salt, and hot sauce. Fold in the cheese. Spoon the mixture into the muffin cups.
4. Bake until the eggs set, about 20 minutes.

Per Serving
calories: 259 | fat: 17g | protein: 24g | carbs: 3g | sugars: 0g | fiber: 0g | sodium: 781mg

Pumpkin Walnut Smoothie Bowl

Prep time: 5 minutes | Cook time: 0 minutes | Serves 2

1 cup plain Greek yogurt
½ cup canned pumpkin purée (not pumpkin pie mix)
1 teaspoon pumpkin pie spice
2 (1-gram) packets stevia
½ teaspoon vanilla extract
Pinch sea salt
½ cup chopped walnuts

1. In a bowl, whisk together the yogurt, pumpkin purée, pumpkin pie spice, stevia, vanilla, and salt (or blend in a blender).
2. Spoon into two bowls. Serve topped with the chopped walnuts.

Per Serving
calories: 292 | fat: 23g | protein: 9g | carbs: 15g | sugars: 6g | fiber: 4g | sodium: 85mg

Quinoa, Teff, and Corn Porridge

Prep time: 5 minutes | Cook time: 35 minutes | Serves 8

1 cup teff
1 cup stone-ground corn grits
1 cup quinoa
¼ teaspoon whole cloves
1 tablespoon
sunflower seed oil
5 cups water
2 cups roughly chopped fresh fruit
2 cups unsalted crushed nuts

1. In an electric pressure cooker, combine the teff, grits, quinoa, and cloves.
2. Add the oil and water, mixing together with a fork.
3. Close and lock the lid, and set the pressure valve to sealing.
4. Select the Porridge setting, and cook for 20 minutes.
5. Once cooking is complete, allow the pressure to release naturally. Carefully remove the lid.
6. Serve each portion with ¼ cup fresh fruit and ¼ cup nuts of your choice.

Per Serving
calories: 417 | fat: 19g | protein: 13g | carbs: 49g | sugars: 5g | fiber: 9g | sodium: 13mg

Ginger Blackberry Bliss Smoothie Bowl

Prep time: 5 minutes | Cook time: 0 minutes | Serves 2

½ cup frozen blackberries
1 cup plain Greek yogurt
1 cup baby spinach
½ cup unsweetened
almond milk
½ teaspoon peeled and grated fresh ginger
¼ cup chopped pecans

1. In a blender or food processor, combine the blackberries, yogurt, spinach, almond milk, and ginger. Blend until smooth.
2. Spoon the mixture into two bowls.
3. Top each bowl with 2 tablespoons of chopped pecans and serve.

Per Serving
calories: 202 | fat: 15g | protein: 7g | carbs: 15g | sugars: 14g | fiber: 4g | sodium: 104mg

Heart-Healthy Yogurt Parfaits

Prep time: 10 minutes | Cook time: 5 minutes | Serves 2

1 cup fresh pineapple chunks
1 cup plain Greek yogurt
¼ cup canned coconut milk
¼ cup flaxseed
2 tablespoons unsweetened toasted coconut flakes
2 tablespoons chopped macadamia nuts

1. Preheat the oven broiler on high.
2. Spread the pineapple chunks in a single layer on a rimmed baking sheet.
3. Broil until the pineapple begins to brown, 4 to 5 minutes.
4. In a small bowl, whisk together the yogurt, coconut milk, and flaxseed. Spoon the mixture into two bowls. Top with the pineapple chunks.
5. Serve with the coconut flakes and chopped macadamia nuts sprinkled over the top.

Per Serving
calories: 402 | fat: 31g | protein: 10g | carbs: 26g | sugars: 16g | fiber: 9g | sodium: 71mg

Avocado Toast with Tomato and Cheese

Prep time: 5 minutes | Cook time: 0 minutes | Serves 2

½ cup cottage cheese
(optional)
½ avocado, mashed
1 teaspoon Dijon mustard
Dash hot sauce

2 slices whole-grain bread, toasted
2 slices tomato

1. In a small bowl, mix together the cottage cheese, avocado, mustard, and hot sauce, if using, until well mixed.
2. Spread the mixture on the toast.
3. Top each piece of toast with a tomato slice.

Per Serving
calories: 179 | fat: 8g | protein: 11g | carbs: 17g | sugars: 5g | fiber: 4g | sodium: 327mg

Coconut Pancakes

Prep time: 5 minutes | Cook time: 15 to 20 minutes | Serves 4

½ cup coconut flour
1 teaspoon baking powder
½ teaspoon ground cinnamon
⅛ teaspoon salt
8 large eggs

⅓ cup unsweetened almond milk
2 tablespoons avocado or coconut oil
1 teaspoon vanilla extract

1. Heat a large skillet over medium-low heat.
2. In a large bowl, whisk together the flour, baking powder, cinnamon, and salt. Set aside.
3. In a medium bowl, whisk together the eggs, almond milk, oil, and vanilla. Pour the wet mixture into the dry ingredients and stir until combined.
4. Pour ⅓ cup of the batter onto the skillet for each pancake. Cook until bubbles appear on the surface of the pancake, about 7 minutes, then flip and cook for 1 minute more.

Per Serving
calories: 270 | fat: 18g | protein: 14g | carbs: 10g | sugars: 2g | fiber: 5g | sodium: 325mg

Blueberry Oat Mini Muffins

Prep time: 12 minutes | Cook time: 10 minutes | Serves 7

½ cup rolled oats
¼ cup whole wheat pastry flour or white whole wheat flour
½ tablespoon baking powder
½ teaspoon ground cardamom or ground cinnamon
⅛ teaspoon kosher salt
2 large eggs

½ cup plain Greek yogurt
2 tablespoons pure maple syrup
2 teaspoons extra-virgin olive oil
½ teaspoon vanilla extract
½ cup frozen blueberries (preferably small wild blueberries)

1. In a large bowl, stir together the oats, flour, baking powder, cardamom, and salt.
2. In a medium bowl, whisk together the eggs, yogurt, maple syrup, oil, and vanilla.
3. Add the egg mixture to oat mixture and stir just until combined. Gently fold in the blueberries.
4. Scoop the batter into each cup of the egg bite mold.
5. Pour 1 cup of water into the electric pressure cooker. Place the egg bite mold on the wire rack and carefully lower it into the pot.
6. Close and lock the lid of the pressure cooker. Set the valve to sealing.
7. Cook on high pressure for 10 minutes.
8. When the cooking is complete, allow the pressure to release naturally for 10 minutes, then quick release any remaining pressure. Hit Cancel.
9. Lift the wire rack out of the pot and place on a cooling rack for 5 minutes. Invert the mold onto the cooling rack to release the muffins.
10. Serve the muffins warm or refrigerate or freeze.

Per Serving
calories: 117 | fat: 4g | protein: 5g | carbs: 15g | sugars: 4g | fiber: 2g | sodium: 89mg

Hoe Cakes

Prep time: 10 minutes | Cook time: 15 minutes | Serves 16 to 18

1 medium egg
½ cup fat-free milk
2 cups cornmeal
3 teaspoons baking powder

1 tablespoon unsalted non-hydrogenated plant-based butter, for greasing the pan

1. In a medium bowl, whisk the egg and milk together.
2. In a separate medium bowl, whisk the cornmeal and baking powder together.
3. Fold the dry ingredients into the wet ingredients until incorporated.
4. In a skillet, melt the butter over medium heat.
5. Add the batter in ¼-cup dollops to the pan (no more than 4 dollops at a time, spaced 1 to 2 inches apart).
6. When the edges become golden brown, turn the cakes, and cook for 30 to 60 seconds more. Repeat until no batter remains.

Per Serving
calories: 69 | fat: 2g | protein: 2g | carbs: 13g | sugars: 1g | fiber: 1g | sodium: 22mg

Breakfast Pita with Egg and Bacon

Prep time: 5 minutes | Cook time: 15 minutes | Serves 2

1 (6-inch) whole-grain pita bread
3 teaspoons extra-virgin olive oil, divided
2 eggs
2 Canadian bacon slices

Juice of ½ lemon
1 cup microgreens
2 tablespoons crumbled goat cheese
Freshly ground black pepper, to taste

1. Heat a large skillet over medium heat. Cut the pita bread in half and brush each side of both halves with ¼ teaspoon of olive oil (using a total of 1 teaspoon oil). Cook for 2 to 3 minutes on each side, then remove from the skillet.
2. In the same skillet, heat 1 teaspoon of oil over medium heat. Crack the eggs into the skillet and cook until the eggs are set, 2 to 3 minutes. Remove from the skillet.

3. In the same skillet, cook the Canadian bacon for 3 to 5 minutes, flipping once.
4. In a large bowl, whisk together the remaining 1 teaspoon of oil and the lemon juice. Add the microgreens and toss to combine.
5. Top each pita half with half of the microgreens, 1 piece of bacon, 1 egg, and 1 tablespoon of goat cheese. Season with pepper and serve.

Per Serving
calories: 251 | fat: 14g | protein: 12g | carbs: 20g | sugars: 1g | fiber: 2g | sodium: 399mg

Breakfast Farro with Berries and Walnuts

Prep time: 8 minutes | Cook time: 10 minutes | Serves 6

1 cup farro, rinsed and drained
1 cup unsweetened almond milk
¼ teaspoon kosher salt
½ teaspoon pure vanilla extract
1 teaspoon ground cinnamon

1 tablespoon pure maple syrup
1½ cups fresh blueberries, raspberries, or strawberries (or a combination)
6 tablespoons chopped walnuts

1. In the electric pressure cooker, combine the farro, almond milk, 1 cup of water, salt, vanilla, cinnamon, and maple syrup.
2. Close and lock the lid. Set the valve to sealing.
3. Cook on high pressure for 10 minutes.
4. When the cooking is complete, allow the pressure to release naturally for 10 minutes, then quick release any remaining pressure. Hit Cancel.
5. Once the pin drops, unlock and remove the lid.
6. Stir the farro. Spoon into bowls and top each serving with ¼ cup of berries and 1 tablespoon of walnuts.

Per Serving (¹/₃ cup)
calories: 189 | fat: 5g | protein: 5g | carbs: 32g | sugars: 6g | fiber: 3g | sodium: 111mg

Tropical Steel Cut Oats

Prep time: 5 minutes | Cook time: 5 minutes | Serves 4

1 cup steel cut oats
1 cup unsweetened almond milk
2 cups coconut water or water
¾ cup frozen chopped peaches
¾ cup frozen mango chunks
1 (2-inch) vanilla bean, scraped (seeds and pod)
Ground cinnamon
¼ cup chopped unsalted macadamia nuts

1. In the electric pressure cooker, combine the oats, almond milk, coconut water, peaches, mango chunks, and vanilla bean seeds and pod. Stir well.
2. Close and lock the lid of the pressure cooker. Set the valve to sealing.
3. Cook on high pressure for 5 minutes.
4. When the cooking is complete, allow the pressure to release naturally for 10 minutes, then quick release any remaining pressure. Hit Cancel.
5. Once the pin drops, unlock and remove the lid.
6. Discard the vanilla bean pod and stir well.
7. Spoon the oats into 4 bowls. Top each serving with a sprinkle of cinnamon and 1 tablespoon of the macadamia nuts.

Per Serving (¾ cup)
calories: 127 | fat: 7g | protein: 2g | carbs: 14g | sugars: 8g | fiber: 3g | sodium: 167mg

Chocolate Zucchini Muffins

Prep time: 15 minutes | Cook time: 20 minutes | Serves 12

1½ cups grated zucchini
1½ cups rolled oats
1 teaspoon ground cinnamon
2 teaspoons baking powder
¼ teaspoon salt
1 large egg
1 teaspoon vanilla extract
¼ cup coconut oil, melted
½ cup unsweetened applesauce
¼ cup honey
¼ cup dark chocolate chips

1. Preheat the oven to 350ºF (180ºC). Grease the cups of a 12-cup muffin tin or line with paper baking liners. Set aside.
2. Place the zucchini in a colander over the sink to drain.
3. In a blender jar, process the oats until they resemble flour. Transfer to a medium mixing bowl and add the cinnamon, baking powder, and salt. Mix well.
4. In another large mixing bowl, combine the egg, vanilla, coconut oil, applesauce, and honey. Stir to combine.
5. Press the zucchini into the colander, draining any liquids, and add to the wet mixture.
6. Stir the dry mixture into the wet mixture, and mix until no dry spots remain. Fold in the chocolate chips.
7. Transfer the batter to the muffin tin, filling each cup a little over halfway. Cook for 16 to 18 minutes until the muffins are lightly browned and a toothpick inserted in the center comes out clean.
8. Store in an airtight container, refrigerated, for up to 5 days.

Per Serving
calories: 121 | fat: 7g | protein: 2g | carbs: 16g | sugars: 7g | fiber: 2g | sodium: 106mg

Hard-boiled Eggs

Prep time: 2 minutes | Cook time: 2 minutes | Serves 9

9 large eggs

1. Pour 1 cup of water into the electric pressure cooker and insert an egg rack. Gently stand the eggs in the rack, fat ends down. If you don't have an egg rack, place the eggs in a steamer basket or on a wire rack.
2. Close and lock the lid of the pressure cooker. Set the valve to sealing.
3. Cook on high pressure for 2 minutes.
4. When the cooking is complete, hit Cancel and allow the pressure to release naturally.
5. Once the pin drops, unlock and remove the lid.
6. Using tongs, carefully remove the eggs from the pressure cooker. Peel or refrigerate the eggs when they are cool enough to handle.

Per Serving
calories: 78 | fat: 5g | protein: 6g | carbs: 1g | sugars: 0g | fiber: 0g | sodium: 62mg

Zucchini Bread

Prep time: 15 minutes | Cook time: 45 minutes | Serves 24

1½ cups gluten-free all-purpose flour
1 cup almond meal
½ cup chickpea flour
1 teaspoon salt
1 teaspoon baking powder
1 teaspoon baking soda
½ teaspoon ground nutmeg
½ teaspoon ground

cinnamon
3 medium brown eggs
¼ cup sunflower seed oil
2 ripe bananas, mashed
2 zucchini, grated, with water squeezed out
2 teaspoons almond extract

1. Preheat the oven to 350ºF (180ºC). Line a 9 × 13-inch pan with parchment paper.
2. In a large bowl, use a fork or whisk to combine the gluten-free flour, almond meal, chickpea flour, salt, baking powder, baking soda, nutmeg, and cinnamon.
3. In a separate large bowl, beat the eggs, oil, bananas, zucchini, and almond extract together well.
4. Fold the dry ingredients into the wet ingredients, stir until well combined, and pour into the prepared pan.
5. Transfer the pan to the oven, and bake for 40 to 45 minutes, or until a butter knife inserted into the center comes out clean. Remove from the oven, and let the bread rest for 15 minutes before serving.

Per Serving
calories: 203 | fat: 11g | protein: 6g | carbs: 21g | sugars: 4g | fiber: 4g | sodium: 323mg

Biscuits

Prep time: 15 minutes | Cook time: 15 minutes | Serves 12

1½ cups gluten-free all-purpose flour
½ cup split pea flour or chickpea flour
½ cup cornmeal
1 teaspoon baking powder
½ teaspoon salt
1 cup low-fat

buttermilk
1 medium egg
2 medium egg whites
4 tablespoons (½ stick) unsalted non-hydrogenated plant-based butter, cold, cut into ¼-inch chunks

1. Preheat the oven to 400ºF (205ºC). Line a rimmed baking sheet with parchment paper.
2. In a medium bowl, whisk the gluten-free flour, split pea flour, cornmeal, baking powder, and salt together.
3. In a large bowl, beat the buttermilk, egg, and egg whites together.
4. Gently fold the dry ingredients into the wet ingredients until just combined, taking care not to overmix.
5. Add the butter to the mixture, gently working together with clean hands. Knead the dough only once or twice.
6. Transfer the dough to a clean workspace, and pat it to a 1-inch thickness.
7. Using a biscuit cutter, cut 12 biscuits, and place them, evenly spaced, onto the prepared baking sheet.
8. Transfer the baking sheet to the oven, and bake for 10 to 15 minutes, or until golden brown.

Per Serving
calories: 133 | fat: 5g | protein: 5g | carbs: 18g | sugars: 2g | fiber: 2g | sodium: 178mg

Toads in Holes

Prep time: 5 minutes | Cook time: 5 minutes | Serves 2

2 tablespoons butter
2 slices whole-wheat bread
2 large eggs

Sea salt and freshly ground black pepper, to taste

1. In a medium nonstick skillet over medium heat, heat the butter until it bubbles.
2. As the butter heats, cut a 3-inch hole in the middle of each piece of bread. Discard the centers.
3. Place the bread pieces in the butter in the pan. Carefully crack an egg into the hole of each piece of bread.
4. Cook until the bread crisps and the egg whites set, about 3 minutes.
5. Flip and cook just until the yolk is almost set, 1 to 2 minutes more.
6. Season to taste with the salt and pepper.

Per Serving
calories: 241 | fat: 17g | protein: 10g | carbs: 12g | sugars: 0g | fiber: 2g | sodium: 307mg

Sausage, Sweet Potato, and Kale Hash

Prep time: 10 minutes | Cook time: 15 minutes | Serves 4

Avocado oil cooking spray
1⅓ cups peeled and diced sweet potatoes
8 cups roughly chopped kale, stemmed and loosely

packed (about 2 bunches)
4 links chicken or turkey breakfast sausage
4 large eggs
4 lemon wedges

1. Heat a large skillet over medium heat. When hot, coat the cooking surface with cooking spray. Cook the sweet potatoes for 4 minutes, stirring once halfway through.
2. Reduce the heat to medium-low and move the potatoes to one side of the skillet. Arrange the kale and sausage in a single layer. Cover and cook for 3 minutes.
3. Stir the vegetables and sausage together, then push them to one side of the skillet to create space for the eggs. Add the eggs and cook them to your liking. Cover the skillet and cook for 3 minutes.
4. Divide the sausage and vegetables into four equal portions and top with an egg and a squeeze of lemon.

Per Serving
calories: 234 | fat: 8g | protein: 12g | carbs: 32g | sugars: 6g | fiber: 5g | sodium: 270mg

Crepe Cakes

Prep time: 5 minutes | Cook time: 20 minutes | Serves 4

Avocado oil cooking spray
4 ounces (113 g) reduced-fat plain cream cheese, softened

2 medium bananas
4 large eggs
½ teaspoon vanilla extract
⅛ teaspoon salt

1. Heat a large skillet over low heat. Coat the cooking surface with cooking spray, and allow the pan to heat for another 2 to 3 minutes.
2. Meanwhile, in a medium bowl, mash the cream cheese and bananas together with a fork until combined. The bananas can be a little chunky.

3. Add the eggs, vanilla, and salt, and mix well.
4. For each cake, drop 2 tablespoons of the batter onto the warmed skillet and use the bottom of a large spoon or ladle to spread it thin. Let it cook for 7 to 9 minutes.
5. Flip the cake over and cook briefly, about 1 minute.

Per Serving
calories: 175 | fat: 9g | protein: 9g | carbs: 15g | sugars: 8g | fiber: 2g | sodium: 213mg

Carrot Oat Pancakes

Prep time: 10 minutes | Cook time: 20 minutes | Serves 4

1 cup rolled oats
1 cup shredded carrots
1 cup low-fat cottage cheese
2 eggs
½ cup unsweetened plain almond milk
1 teaspoon baking powder

½ teaspoon ground cinnamon
2 tablespoons ground flaxseed
¼ cup plain nonfat Greek yogurt
1 tablespoon pure maple syrup
2 teaspoons canola oil, divided

1. In a blender jar, process the oats until they resemble flour. Add the carrots, cottage cheese, eggs, almond milk, baking powder, cinnamon, and flaxseed to the jar. Process until smooth.
2. In a small bowl, combine the yogurt and maple syrup and stir well. Set aside.
3. In a large skillet, heat 1 teaspoon of oil over medium heat. Using a measuring cup, add ¼ cup of batter per pancake to the skillet. Cook for 1 to 2 minutes until bubbles form on the surface, and flip the pancakes. Cook for another minute until the pancakes are browned and cooked through. Repeat with the remaining 1 teaspoon of oil and remaining batter.
4. Serve warm topped with the maple yogurt.

Per Serving
calories: 227 | fat: 8g | protein: 14g | carbs: 24g | sugars: 6g | fiber: 4g | sodium: 402mg

Cranberry Almond Grits

Prep time: 10 minutes | Cook time: 10 minutes | Serves 5

¾ cup stone-ground grits or polenta (not instant)
½ cup unsweetened dried cranberries
Pinch kosher salt
1 tablespoon unsalted

butter or ghee (optional)
1 tablespoon half-and-half
¼ cup sliced almonds, toasted

1. In the electric pressure cooker, stir together the grits, cranberries, salt, and 3 cups of water.
2. Close and lock the lid. Set the valve to sealing.
3. Cook on high pressure for 10 minutes.
4. When the cooking is complete, hit Cancel and quick release the pressure.
5. Once the pin drops, unlock and remove the lid.
6. Add the butter (if using) and half-and-half. Stir until the mixture is creamy, adding more half-and-half if necessary.
7. Spoon into serving bowls and sprinkle with almonds.

Per Serving (½ cup)
calories: 218 | fat: 10g | protein: 5g | carbs: 32g | sugars: 7g | fiber: 4g | sodium: 28mg

Broccoli and Mushroom Frittata

Prep time: 5 minutes | Cook time: 10 minutes | Serves 4

2 tablespoons extra-virgin olive oil
½ onion, finely chopped
1 cup broccoli florets
1 cup sliced shiitake

mushrooms
1 garlic clove, minced
8 large eggs, beaten
½ teaspoon sea salt
½ cup grated Parmesan cheese

1. Preheat the oven broiler on high.
2. In a medium ovenproof skillet over medium-high heat, heat the olive oil until it shimmers.
3. Add the onion, broccoli, and mushrooms, and cook, stirring occasionally, until the vegetables start to brown, about 5 minutes. Add the garlic and cook, stirring constantly, for 30 seconds. Arrange the vegetables in an even layer on the bottom of the pan.

4. While the vegetables cook, in a small bowl, whisk together the eggs and salt. Carefully pour the eggs over the vegetables. Cook without stirring, allowing the eggs to set around the vegetables. As the eggs begin to set around the edges, use a spatula to pull the edges away from the sides of the pan. Tilt the pan and allow the uncooked eggs to run into the spaces. Cook 1 to 2 minutes more, until it sets around the edges. The eggs will still be runny on top.
5. Sprinkle with the Parmesan and place the pan in the broiler. Broil until brown and puffy, about 3 minutes.
6. Cut into wedges to serve.

Per Serving
calories: 280 | fat: 21g | protein: 19g | carbs: 7g | sugars: 1g | fiber: 2g | sodium: 654mg

Orange Muffins

Prep time: 15 minutes | Cook time: 15 minutes | Serves 9

2½ cups finely ground almond flour
¾ teaspoon ground cinnamon
½ teaspoon baking powder
½ teaspoon ground cardamom
¼ teaspoon salt
4 tablespoons

avocado or coconut oil
2 large eggs
Grated zest and juice of 1 medium orange
1 tablespoon raw honey or 100% pure maple syrup
¼ teaspoon vanilla extract

1. Preheat the oven to 375ºF (190ºC).
2. In a large bowl, whisk together the almond flour, cinnamon, baking powder, cardamom, and salt. Set aside.
3. In a medium bowl, whisk together the oil, eggs, zest, juice, honey, and vanilla. Add this mixture to the dry ingredients, and stir until well combined.
4. In a nonstick muffin tin, fill each muffin cup until nearly full.
5. Bake for 15 minutes, or until the top center is firm.

Per Serving
calories: 288 | fat: 23g | protein: 8g | carbs: 16g | sugars: 10g | fiber: 4g | sodium: 97mg

Low-Carb Peanut Butter Pancakes

Prep time: 10 minutes | Cook time: 10 minutes | Serves 2

1 cup almond flour	(plain, unsweetened)
½ teaspoon baking soda	2 tablespoons canola oil, plus more for cooking
Pinch sea salt	
2 large eggs	4 tablespoons peanut butter
¼ cup sparkling water	

1. Heat a nonstick griddle over medium-high heat.
2. In a small bowl, whisk together the almond flour, baking soda, and salt.
3. In a glass measuring cup, whisk together the eggs, water, and oil.
4. Pour the liquid ingredients into the dry ingredients, and mix gently until just combined.
5. Brush a small amount of canola oil onto the griddle.
6. Using all of the batter, spoon four pancakes onto the griddle.
7. Cook until set on one side, about 3 minutes. Flip with a spatula and continue cooking on the other side.
8. Before serving, spread each pancake with 1 tablespoon of the peanut butter.

Per Serving

calories: 454 | fat: 41g | protein: 17g | carbs: 8g | sugars: 3g | fiber: 3g | sodium: 408mg

Brussels Sprouts and Egg Scramble

Prep time: 5 minutes | Cook time: 20 minutes | Serves 4

Avocado oil cooking spray	halved lengthwise
4 slices low-sodium turkey bacon	8 large eggs
20 Brussels sprouts,	¼ cup crumbled feta, for garnish

1. Heat a large skillet over medium heat. When hot, coat the cooking surface with cooking spray and cook the bacon to your liking.
2. Carefully remove the bacon from the pan and set it on a plate lined with a paper towel to drain and cool.
3. Place the Brussels sprouts in the skillet cut-side down, and cook for 3 minutes.

4. Reduce the heat to medium-low. Flip the Brussels sprouts, move them to one side of the skillet, and cover. Cook for another 3 minutes.
5. Uncover. Cook the eggs to over-medium alongside the Brussels sprouts, or to your liking.
6. Crumble the bacon once it has cooled.
7. Divide the Brussels sprouts into 4 portions and top each portion with one-quarter of the crumbled bacon and 2 eggs. Add 1 tablespoon of feta to each portion.

Per Serving

calories: 253 | fat: 15g | protein: 21g | carbs: 10g | sugars: 4g | fiber: 4g | sodium: 343mg

Veggie and Egg White Scramble

Prep time: 5 minutes | Cook time: 10 minutes | Serves 2

2 tablespoons extra-virgin olive oil	4 whole large eggs), beaten
½ red onion, finely chopped	½ teaspoon sea salt
1 green bell pepper, seeded and finely chopped	2 ounces (57 g) grated pepper Jack cheese
8 large egg whites (or	Salsa (optional, for serving)

1. In a medium nonstick skillet over medium-high heat, heat the olive oil until it shimmers.
2. Add the onion and bell pepper and cook, stirring occasionally, until the vegetables begin to brown, about 5 minutes.
3. Meanwhile, in a small bowl, whisk together the egg whites and salt.
4. Add the egg whites to the pan and cook, stirring, until the whites set, about 3 minutes. Add the cheese. Cook, stirring, 1 minute more.
5. Serve topped with salsa, if desired.

Per Serving

calories: 314 | fat: 23g | protein: 22g | carbs: 6g | sugars: 3g | fiber: 1g | sodium: 977mg

Tofu, Kale, and Mushroom Breakfast Scramble

Prep time: 5 minutes | Cook time: 10 minutes | Serves 2

2 tablespoons extra-virgin olive oil
½ red onion, finely chopped
8 ounces (227 g) mushrooms, sliced
1 cup chopped kale
8 ounces (227 g)

tofu, cut into pieces
2 garlic cloves, minced
Pinch red pepper flakes
½ teaspoon sea salt
⅛ teaspoon freshly ground black pepper

1. In a medium nonstick skillet over medium-high heat, heat the olive oil until it shimmers.
2. Add the onion, mushrooms, and kale. Cook, stirring occasionally, until the vegetables begin to brown, about 5 minutes.
3. Add the tofu. Cook, stirring, until the tofu starts to brown, 3 to 4 minutes more.
4. Add the garlic, red pepper flakes, salt, and pepper. Cook, stirring constantly, for 30 seconds more.

Per Serving

calories: 234 | fat: 16g | protein: 13g | carbs: 12g | sugars: 4g | fiber: 2g | sodium: 673mg

Smoked Salmon and Asparagus Quiche Cups

Prep time: 15 minutes | Cook time: 15 minutes | Serves 2

Nonstick cooking spray
4 asparagus spears, cut into ½-inch pieces
2 tablespoons finely chopped onion
3 ounces (85 g) smoked salmon

(skinless and boneless), chopped
3 large eggs
2 tablespoons 2% milk
¼ teaspoon dried dill
Pinch ground white pepper

1. Pour 1½ cups of water into the electric pressure cooker and insert a wire rack or trivet.
2. Lightly spray the bottom and sides of the ramekins with nonstick cooking spray. Divide the asparagus, onion, and salmon between the ramekins.
3. In a measuring cup with a spout, whisk together the eggs, milk, dill, and white pepper. Pour half of the egg mixture into each ramekin. Loosely cover the ramekins with aluminum foil.
4. Carefully place the ramekins inside the pot on the rack.
5. Close and lock the lid of the pressure cooker. Set the valve to sealing.
6. Cook on high pressure for 15 minutes.
7. When the cooking is complete, hit Cancel and quick release the pressure.
8. Once the pin drops, unlock and remove the lid.
9. Carefully remove the ramekins from the pot. Cool, covered, for 5 minutes.
10. Run a small silicone spatula or a knife around the edge of each ramekin. Invert each quiche onto a small plate and serve.

Per Serving

calories: 180 | fat: 9g | protein: 20g | carbs: 3g | sugars: 1g | fiber: 1g | sodium: 646mg

Sausage and Pepper Breakfast Burrito

Prep time: 10 minutes | Cook time: 15 minutes | Serves 4

8 ounces (227 g) bulk pork breakfast sausage
½ onion, chopped
1 green bell pepper, seeded and chopped
8 large eggs, beaten
4 (6-inch) low-carb

tortillas
1 cup shredded pepper Jack cheese
½ cup sour cream (optional, for serving)
½ cup prepared salsa (optional, for serving)

1. In a large nonstick skillet on medium-high heat, cook the sausage, crumbling it with a spoon, until browned, about 5 minutes. Add the onion and bell pepper. Cook, stirring, until the veggies are soft, about 3 minutes. Add the eggs and cook, stirring, until eggs are set, about 3 minutes more.
2. Spoon the egg mixture onto the 4 tortillas. Top each with the cheese and fold into a burrito shape.
3. Serve with sour cream and salsa, if desired.

Per Serving

calories: 485 | fat: 36g | protein: 32g | carbs: 13g | sugars: 3g | fiber: 8g | sodium: 810mg

Gouda Egg Casserole with Canadian Bacon

Prep time: 12 minutes | Cook time: 20 minutes | Serves 4

Nonstick cooking spray
1 slice whole grain bread, toasted
½ cup shredded smoked Gouda cheese
3 slices Canadian bacon, chopped
6 large eggs
¼ cup half-and-half
¼ teaspoon kosher salt
¼ teaspoon freshly ground black pepper
¼ teaspoon dry mustard

1. Spray a 6-inch cake pan with cooking spray, or if the pan is nonstick, skip this step. If you don't have a 6-inch cake pan, any bowl or pan that fits inside your pressure cooker should work.
2. Crumble the toast into the bottom of the pan. Sprinkle with the cheese and Canadian bacon.
3. In a medium bowl, whisk together the eggs, half-and-half, salt, pepper, and dry mustard.
4. Pour the egg mixture into the pan. Loosely cover the pan with aluminum foil.
5. Pour 1½ cups water into the electric pressure cooker and insert a wire rack or trivet. Place the covered pan on top of the rack.
6. Close and lock the lid of the pressure cooker. Set the valve to sealing.
7. Cook on high pressure for 20 minutes.
8. When the cooking is complete, hit Cancel and quick release the pressure.
9. Once the pin drops, unlock and remove the lid.
10. Carefully transfer the pan from the pressure cooker to a cooling rack and let it sit for 5 minutes.
11. Cut into 4 wedges and serve.

Per Serving
calories: 247 | fat: 15g | protein: 20g | carbs: 8g | sugars: 1g | fiber: 1g | sodium: 717mg

Breakfast Tacos

Prep time: 5 minutes | Cook time: 10 minutes | Serves 4

Taco Filling:
Avocado oil cooking spray
1 medium green bell pepper, chopped
8 large eggs
¼ cup shredded sharp Cheddar cheese
4 (6-inch) whole-
Pico De Gallo:
1 tomato, diced
½ large white onion, diced
2 tablespoons chopped fresh cilantro
½ jalapeño pepper,
wheat tortillas
1 cup fresh spinach leaves
½ cup Pico de Gallo
Scallions, chopped, for garnish (optional)
Avocado slices, for garnish (optional)

stemmed, seeded, and diced
1 tablespoon freshly squeezed lime juice
⅛ teaspoon salt

Make the Taco Filling
1. Heat a medium skillet over medium-low heat. When hot, coat the cooking surface with cooking spray and put the pepper in the skillet. Cook for 4 minutes.
2. Meanwhile, whisk the eggs in a medium bowl, then add the cheese and whisk to combine. Pour the eggs and cheese into the skillet with the green peppers and scramble until the eggs are fully cooked, about 5 minutes.
3. Microwave the tortillas very briefly, about 8 seconds.
4. For each serving, top a tortilla with one-quarter of the spinach, eggs, and pico de gallo. Garnish with scallions and avocado slices (if using).

Make the Pico De Gallo
1. In a medium bowl, combine the tomato, onion, cilantro, pepper, lime juice, and salt. Mix well and serve.

Per Serving
calories: 276 | fat: 12g | protein: 16g | carbs: 28g | sugars: 8g | fiber: 3g | sodium: 562mg

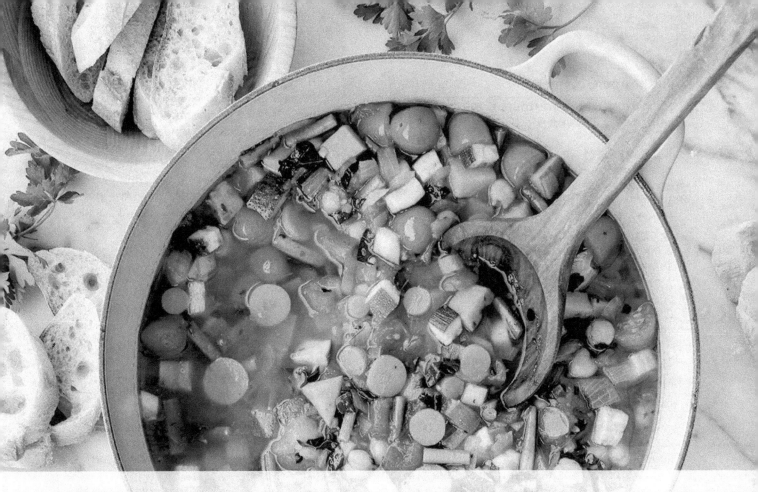

Chapter 3 Soups and Stews

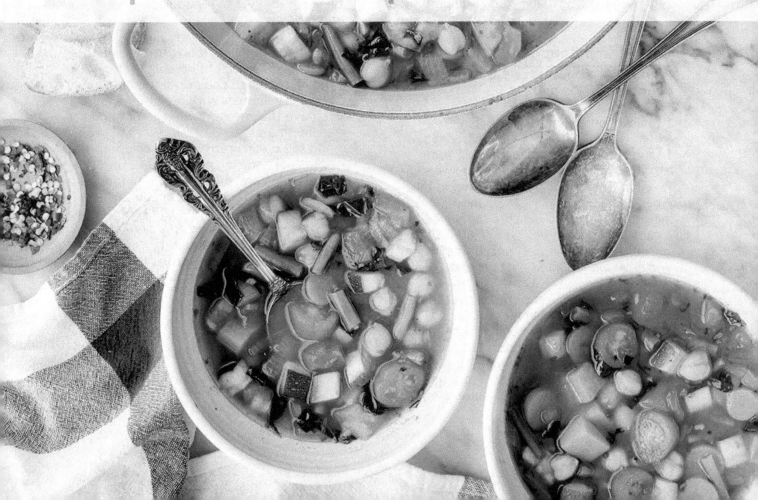

Authentic Gazpacho

Prep time: 15 minutes | Cook time: 0 minutes | Serves 4

3 pounds (1.4 kg) ripe tomatoes, chopped
1 cup low-sodium tomato juice
½ red onion, chopped
1 cucumber, peeled, seeded, and chopped
1 red bell pepper, seeded and chopped
2 celery stalks, chopped

2 tablespoons chopped fresh parsley
2 garlic cloves, chopped
2 tablespoons extra-virgin olive oil
2 tablespoons red wine vinegar
1 teaspoon honey
½ teaspoon salt
¼ teaspoon freshly ground black pepper

1. In a blender jar, combine the tomatoes, tomato juice, onion, cucumber, bell pepper, celery, parsley, garlic, olive oil, vinegar, honey, salt, and pepper. Pulse until blended but still slightly chunky.
2. Adjust the seasonings as needed and serve.
3. To store, transfer to a nonreactive, airtight container and refrigerate for up to 3 days.

Per Serving
calories: 170 | fat: 8g | protein: 5g | carbs: 24g | sugars: 16g | fiber: 6g | sodium: 332mg

Thai Shrimp Soup

Prep time: 10 minutes | Cook time: 10 minutes | Serves 4

1 tablespoon coconut oil
1 tablespoon Thai red curry paste
½ onion, sliced
3 garlic cloves, minced
2 cups chopped carrots
½ cup whole unsalted

peanuts
4 cups low-sodium vegetable broth
½ cup unsweetened plain almond milk
½ pound (227 g) shrimp, peeled and deveined
Minced fresh cilantro, for garnish

1. In a large pan, heat the oil over medium-high heat until shimmering.
2. Add the curry paste and cook, stirring constantly, for 1 minute. Add the onion, garlic, carrots, and peanuts to the pan, and continue to cook for 2 to 3 minutes until the onion begins to soften.

3. Add the broth and bring to a boil. Reduce the heat to low and simmer for 5 to 6 minutes until the carrots are tender.
4. Using an immersion blender or in a blender, purée the soup until smooth and return it to the pot. With the heat still on low, add the almond milk and stir to combine. Add the shrimp to the pot and cook for 2 to 3 minutes until cooked through.
5. Garnish with cilantro and serve.

Per Serving
calories: 237 | fat: 14g | protein: 14g | carbs: 17g | sugars: 6g | fiber: 5g | sodium: 619mg

Chicken Zoodle Soup

Prep time: 10 minutes | Cook time: 15 minutes | Serves 4

2 tablespoons extra-virgin olive oil
12 ounces (340 g) chicken breast, chopped
1 onion, chopped
2 carrots, chopped
2 celery stalks, chopped
2 garlic cloves

6 cups unsalted chicken broth
1 teaspoon dried thyme
1 teaspoon sea salt
2 medium zucchinis, cut into noodles (or store-bought zucchini noodles)

1. In a large pot over medium-high heat, heat the olive oil until it shimmers. Add the chicken and cook until it is opaque, about 5 minutes. With a slotted spoon, remove the chicken from the pot and set aside on a plate.
2. Add the onion, carrots, and celery to the pot. Cook, stirring occasionally, until the vegetables are soft, about 5 minutes. Add the garlic and cook, stirring constantly, for 30 seconds. Add the chicken broth, thyme, and salt. Bring to a boil, and reduce the heat to medium.
3. Add the zucchini and return the chicken to the pan, adding any juices that have collected on the plate. Cook, stirring occasionally, until the zucchini noodles are soft, 1 to 2 minutes more.

Per Serving
calories: 236 | fat: 10g | protein: 27g | carbs: 11g | sugars: 4g | fiber: 3g | sodium: 201mg

Quick Clam Chowder

Prep time: 10 minutes | Cook time: 15 minutes | Serves 4

2 tablespoons extra-virgin olive oil
3 slices pepper bacon, chopped
1 onion, chopped
1 red bell pepper, seeded and chopped
1 fennel bulb, chopped
3 tablespoons flour
5 cups low-sodium or unsalted chicken broth
6 ounces (170 g) chopped canned clams, undrained
½ teaspoon sea salt
½ cup milk

1. In a large pot over medium-high heat, heat the olive oil until it shimmers. Add the bacon and cook, stirring, until browned, about 4 minutes. Remove the bacon from the fat with a slotted spoon, and set it aside on a plate.
2. Add the onion, bell pepper, and fennel to the fat in the pot. Cook, stirring occasionally, until the vegetables are soft, about 5 minutes. Add the flour and cook, stirring constantly, for 1 minute. Add the broth, clams, and salt. Bring to a simmer. Cook, stirring, until the soup thickens, about 5 minutes more.
3. Stir in the milk and return the bacon to the pot. Cook, stirring, 1 minute more.

Per Serving
calories: 335 | fat: 20g | protein: 20g | carbs: 21g | sugars: 6g | fiber: 3g | sodium: 496mg

Cauliflower Leek Soup

Prep time: 10 minutes | Cook time: 20 minutes | Serves 2

Avocado oil cooking spray
2½ cups chopped leeks (2 to 3 leeks)
2½ cups cauliflower florets
1 garlic clove, peeled
1/3 cup low-sodium vegetable broth
½ cup half-and-half
¼ teaspoon salt
¼ teaspoon freshly ground black pepper

1. Heat a large stockpot over medium-low heat. When hot, coat the cooking surface with cooking spray. Put the leeks and cauliflower into the pot.
2. Increase the heat to medium and cover the pan. Cook for 10 minutes, stirring halfway through.
3. Add the garlic and cook for 5 minutes.
4. Add the broth and deglaze the pan, stirring to scrape up the browned bits from the bottom.
5. Transfer the broth and vegetables to a food processor or blender and add the half-and-half, salt, and pepper. Blend well.

Per Serving
calories: 173 | fat: 7g | protein: 6g | carbs: 24g | sugars: 8g | fiber: 5g | sodium: 487mg

Zucchini Soup with Roasted Chickpeas

Prep time: 10 minutes | Cook time: 20 minutes | Serves 4

1 (15-ounce / 425-g) can low-sodium chickpeas, drained and rinsed
1 teaspoon extra-virgin olive oil, plus 1 tablespoon
¼ teaspoon smoked paprika
Pinch salt, plus ½ teaspoon
3 medium zucchini, coarsely chopped
3 cups low-sodium vegetable broth
½ onion, diced
3 garlic cloves, minced
2 tablespoons plain low-fat Greek yogurt
Freshly ground black pepper, to taste

1. Preheat the oven to 425ºF (220ºC). Line a baking sheet with parchment paper.
2. In a medium mixing bowl, toss the chickpeas with 1 teaspoon of olive oil, the smoked paprika, and a pinch salt. Transfer to the prepared baking sheet and roast until crispy, about 20 minutes, stirring once. Set aside.
3. Meanwhile, in a medium pot, heat the remaining 1 tablespoon of oil over medium heat.
4. Add the zucchini, broth, onion, and garlic to the pot, and bring to a boil. Reduce the heat to a simmer, and cook until the zucchini and onion are tender, about 20 minutes.
5. In a blender jar, or using an immersion blender, purée the soup. Return to the pot.
6. Add the yogurt, remaining ½ teaspoon of salt, and pepper, and stir well. Serve topped with the roasted chickpeas.

Per Serving
calories: 189 | fat: 7g | protein: 8g | carbs: 24g | sugars: 7g | fiber: 7g | sodium: 527mg

Split Pea Soup with Carrots

Prep time: 8 minutes | Cook time: 15 minutes | Serves 4

1½ cups dried green split peas, rinsed and drained
4 cups vegetable broth or water
2 celery stalks, chopped
1 medium onion, chopped
2 carrots, chopped
3 garlic cloves, minced
1 teaspoon herbes de Provence
1 teaspoon liquid smoke
Kosher salt and freshly ground black pepper, to taste
Shredded carrot, for garnish (optional)

1. In the electric pressure cooker, combine the peas, broth, celery, onion, carrots, garlic, herbes de Provence, and liquid smoke.
2. Close and lock the lid of the pressure cooker. Set the valve to sealing.
3. Cook on high pressure for 15 minutes.
4. When the cooking is complete, hit Cancel and allow the pressure to release naturally for 10 minutes, then quick release any remaining pressure.
5. Once the pin drops, unlock and remove the lid.
6. Stir the soup and season with salt and pepper.
7. Spoon into serving bowls and sprinkle shredded carrots on top (if using).

Per Serving (1¼ cups)
calories: 284 | fat: 1g | protein: 19g | carbs: 52g | sugars: 9g | fiber: 21g | sodium: 60mg

Curried Carrot and Coconut Soup

Prep time: 10 minutes | Cook time: 5 minutes | Serves 6

1 tablespoon extra-virgin olive oil
1 small onion, coarsely chopped
2 celery stalks, coarsely chopped
1½ teaspoons curry powder
1 teaspoon ground cumin
1 teaspoon minced fresh ginger
6 medium carrots, roughly chopped
4 cups low-sodium vegetable broth
¼ teaspoon salt
1 cup canned coconut milk
¼ teaspoon freshly ground black pepper
1 tablespoon chopped fresh cilantro

1. Heat an Instant Pot to high and add the olive oil.
2. Sauté the onion and celery for 2 to 3 minutes. Add the curry powder, cumin, and ginger to the pot and cook until fragrant, about 30 seconds.
3. Add the carrots, vegetable broth, and salt to the pot. Close and seal, and set for 5 minutes on high. Allow the pressure to release naturally.
4. In a blender jar, carefully purée the soup in batches and transfer back to the pot.
5. Stir in the coconut milk and pepper, and heat through. Top with the cilantro and serve.

Per Serving
calories: 145 | fat: 11g | protein: 2g | carbs: 13g | sugars: 4g | fiber: 3g | sodium: 238mg

Taco Soup

Prep time: 5 minutes | Cook time: 20 minutes | Serves 4

Avocado oil cooking spray
1 medium red bell pepper, chopped
½ cup chopped yellow onion
1 pound (454 g) 93% lean ground beef
1 teaspoon ground cumin
½ teaspoon salt
½ teaspoon chili powder
½ teaspoon garlic powder
2 cups low-sodium beef broth
1 (15-ounce / 425-g) can no-salt-added diced tomatoes
1½ cups frozen corn
⅓ cup half-and-half

1. Heat a large stockpot over medium-low heat. When hot, coat the cooking surface with cooking spray. Put the pepper and onion in the pan and cook for 5 minutes.
2. Add the ground beef, cumin, salt, chili powder, and garlic powder. Cook for 5 to 7 minutes, stirring and breaking apart the beef as needed.
3. Add the broth, diced tomatoes with their juices, and corn. Increase the heat to medium-high and simmer for 10 minutes.
4. Remove from the heat and stir in the half-and-half.

Per Serving
calories: 320 | fat: 12g | protein: 30g | carbs: 23g | sugars: 7g | fiber: 4g | sodium: 456mg

Lentil Vegetable Soup

Prep time: 10 minutes | Cook time: 15 minutes | Serves 4

2 tablespoons extra-virgin olive oil
1 onion, finely chopped
1 carrot, chopped
1 cup chopped kale (stems removed)
3 garlic cloves, minced
1 cup canned lentils, drained and rinsed
5 cups unsalted vegetable broth
2 teaspoons dried rosemary (or 1 tablespoon chopped fresh rosemary)
½ teaspoon sea salt
¼ teaspoon freshly ground black pepper

1. In a large pot over medium-high heat, heat the olive oil until it shimmers. Add the onion and carrot and cook, stirring, until the vegetables begin to soften, about 3 minutes. Add the kale and cook for 3 minutes more. Add the garlic and cook, stirring constantly, for 30 seconds.
2. Stir in the lentils, vegetable broth, rosemary, salt, and pepper. Bring to a simmer. Simmer, stirring occasionally, for 5 minutes more.

Per Serving

calories: 160 | fat: 7g | protein: 6g | carbs: 19g | sugars: 12g | fiber: 6g | sodium: 187mg

Moroccan Eggplant Stew

Prep time: 20 minutes | Cook time: 3 minutes | Serves 4

2 tablespoons avocado oil
1 large onion, minced
2 garlic cloves, minced
1 teaspoon ras el hanout spice blend or curry powder
¼ teaspoon cayenne pepper
1 teaspoon kosher salt
1 cup vegetable broth or water
1 tablespoon tomato paste
2 cups chopped eggplant
2 medium gold potatoes, peeled and chopped
4 ounces (113 g) tomatillos, husks removed, chopped
1 (14-ounce / 397-g) can diced tomatoes

1. Set the electric pressure cooker to the Sauté setting. When the pot is hot, pour in the avocado oil.

2. Sauté the onion for 3 to 5 minutes, until it begins to soften. Add the garlic, ras el hanout, cayenne, and salt. Cook and stir for about 30 seconds. Hit Cancel.
3. Stir in the broth and tomato paste. Add the eggplant, potatoes, tomatillos, and tomatoes with their juices.
4. Close and lock the lid of the pressure cooker. Set the valve to sealing.
5. Cook on high pressure for 3 minutes.
6. When the cooking is complete, hit Cancel and allow the pressure to release naturally.
7. Once the pin drops, unlock and remove the lid.
8. Stir well and spoon into serving bowls.

Per Serving (1½ cups)

calories: 216 | fat: 8g | protein: 4g | carbs: 28g | sugars: 9g | fiber: 8g | sodium: 735mg

Tomato Kale Soup

Prep time: 10 minutes | Cook time: 15 minutes | Serves 4

1 tablespoon extra-virgin olive oil
1 medium onion, chopped
2 carrots, finely chopped
3 garlic cloves, minced
4 cups low-sodium vegetable broth
1 (28-ounce / 794-g) can crushed tomatoes
½ teaspoon dried oregano
¼ teaspoon dried basil
4 cups chopped baby kale leaves
¼ teaspoon salt

1. In a large pot, heat the oil over medium heat. Add the onion and carrots to the pan. Sauté for 3 to 5 minutes until they begin to soften. Add the garlic and sauté for 30 seconds more, until fragrant.
2. Add the vegetable broth, tomatoes, oregano, and basil to the pot and bring to a boil. Reduce the heat to low and simmer for 5 minutes.
3. Using an immersion blender, purée the soup.
4. Add the kale and simmer for 3 more minutes. Season with the salt. Serve immediately.

Per Serving

calories: 172 | fat: 5g | protein: 6g | carbs: 30g | sugars: 13g | fiber: 8g | sodium: 601mg

Slow Cooker Chicken and Vegetable Soup

Prep time: 10 minutes | Cook time: 4 hours | Serves 4

1 medium potato, peeled and chopped into 1-inch pieces
3 celery stalks, chopped into 1-inch pieces
2 cups chopped baby carrots
1 cup chopped white onion
2 cups chopped green beans
2 cups low-sodium chicken broth
2 tablespoons tomato paste
2 tablespoons Italian seasoning
1 pound (454 g) boneless, skinless chicken breasts, chopped
Freshly ground black pepper, to taste

1. Put the potato, celery, carrots, onion, green beans, broth, tomato paste, Italian seasoning, and chicken into a slow cooker and cook on high for 4 hours.
2. Season with freshly ground black pepper.

Per Serving
calories: 232 | fat: 3g | protein: 30g | carbs: 25g | sugars: 7g | fiber: 6g | sodium: 180mg

Cheeseburger Soup

Prep time: 5 minutes | Cook time: 25 minutes | Serves 4

Avocado oil cooking spray
½ cup diced white onion
½ cup diced celery
½ cup sliced portobello mushrooms
1 pound (454 g) 93%
lean ground beef
1 (15-ounce / 425-g) can no-salt-added diced tomatoes
2 cups low-sodium beef broth
⅓ cup half-and-half
¾ cup shredded sharp Cheddar cheese

1. Heat a large stockpot over medium-low heat. When hot, coat the cooking surface with cooking spray. Put the onion, celery, and mushrooms into the pot. Cook for 7 minutes, stirring occasionally.
2. Add the ground beef and cook for 5 minutes, stirring and breaking apart as needed.
3. Add the diced tomatoes with their juices and the broth. Increase the heat to medium-high and simmer for 10 minutes.
4. Remove the pot from the heat and stir in the half-and-half.
5. Serve topped with the cheese.

Per Serving
calories: 330 | fat: 18g | protein: 33g | carbs: 9g | sugars: 5g | fiber: 2g | sodium: 321mg

Lime Chicken Tortilla Soup

Prep time: 10 minutes | Cook time: 35 minutes | Serves 4

1 tablespoon extra-virgin olive oil
1 onion, thinly sliced
1 garlic clove, minced
1 jalapeño pepper, diced
2 boneless, skinless chicken breasts
4 cups low-sodium chicken broth
1 Roma tomato, diced
½ teaspoon salt
2 (6-inch) corn tortillas, cut into thin strips
Nonstick cooking spray
Juice of 1 lime
Minced fresh cilantro, for garnish
¼ cup shredded Cheddar cheese, for garnish

1. In a medium pot, heat the oil over medium-high heat. Add the onion and cook for 3 to 5 minutes until it begins to soften. Add the garlic and jalapeño, and cook until fragrant, about 1 minute more.
2. Add the chicken, chicken broth, tomato, and salt to the pot and bring to a boil. Reduce the heat to medium and simmer gently for 20 to 25 minutes until the chicken breasts are cooked through. Remove the chicken from the pot and set aside.
3. Preheat a broiler to high.
4. Spray the tortilla strips with nonstick cooking spray and toss to coat. Spread in a single layer on a baking sheet and broil for 3 to 5 minutes, flipping once, until crisp.
5. When the chicken is cool enough to handle, shred it with two forks and return to the pot.
6. Season the soup with the lime juice. Serve hot, garnished with cilantro, cheese, and tortilla strips.

Per Serving
calories: 191 | fat: 8g | protein: 19g | carbs: 13g | sugars: 2g | fiber: 2g | sodium: 482mg

Sweet Potato and Pumpkin Soup

Prep time: 10 minutes | Cook time: 45 minutes | Serves 8 to 10

3 cups vegetable broth, divided
1 celery stalk, roughly chopped
1 cup roughly chopped tomato
1 red bell pepper, chopped
1 large sweet potato, peeled and cut into

2-inch cubes
1 small pumpkin, peeled and cut into 2-inch cubes
1 bay leaf
1 teaspoon paprika
2 cups roasted unsalted peanuts
Baby sage leaves (optional)

1. In a large Dutch oven, bring 1 cup of broth to a simmer over medium heat.
2. Add the celery, tomato, and bell pepper and cook for 5 to 7 minutes, or until softened.
3. Add the sweet potato, pumpkin, bay leaf, paprika, and the remaining 2 cups of broth. Cover and cook for 30 minutes, or until the sweet potato and pumpkin are soft.
4. Add the peanuts and cook for 5 minutes, or until the peanuts become less crunchy. Discard the bay leaf.
5. Transfer to a heat-safe blender, and pulse until the soup has a batter-like consistency.
6. Serve and garnish with baby sage leaves.

Per Serving

calories: 266 | fat: 18g | protein: 12g | carbs: 19g | sugars: 6g | fiber: 5g | sodium: 50mg

Vegetable Beef Soup

Prep time: 10 minutes | Cook time: 15 minutes | Serves 4

1 pound (454 g) ground beef
1 onion, chopped
2 celery stalks, chopped
1 carrot, chopped
1 teaspoon dried

rosemary
6 cups low-sodium beef or chicken broth
½ teaspoon sea salt
⅛ teaspoon freshly ground black pepper
2 cups peas

1. In a large pot over medium-high heat, cook the ground beef, crumbling with the side of a spoon, until browned, about 5 minutes.
2. Add the onion, celery, carrot, and rosemary. Cook, stirring occasionally, until the vegetables start to soften, about 5 minutes.
3. Add the broth, salt, pepper, and peas. Bring to a simmer. Reduce the heat and simmer, stirring, until warmed through, about 5 minutes more.

Per Serving

calories: 355 | fat: 17g | protein: 34g | carbs: 18g | sugars: 6g | fiber: 5g | sodium: 362mg

Spiced Lamb Stew

Prep time: 20 minutes | Cook time: 2 hours 15 minutes | Serves 4

2 tablespoons extra-virgin olive oil
1½ pounds (680 g) lamb shoulder, cut into 1-inch chunks
½ sweet onion, chopped
1 tablespoon grated fresh ginger
2 teaspoons minced garlic
1 teaspoon ground cinnamon
1 teaspoon ground

cumin
¼ teaspoon ground cloves
2 sweet potatoes, peeled, diced
2 cups low-sodium beef broth
Sea salt and freshly ground back pepper, to taste
2 teaspoons chopped fresh parsley, for garnish

1. Preheat the oven to 300ºF (150ºC).
2. Place a large ovenproof skillet over medium-high heat and add the olive oil.
3. Brown the lamb, stirring occasionally, for about 6 minutes.
4. Add the onion, ginger, garlic, cinnamon, cumin, and cloves, and sauté for 5 minutes.
5. Add the sweet potatoes and beef broth and bring the stew to a boil.
6. Cover the skillet and transfer the lamb to the oven. Braise, stirring occasionally, until the lamb is very tender, about 2 hours.
7. Remove the stew from the oven and season with salt and pepper.
8. Serve garnished with the parsley.

Per Serving

calories: 544 | fat: 35g | protein: 32g | carbs: 16g | sugars: 4g | fiber: 2g | sodium: 395mg

Red Lentil Soup

Prep time: 10 minutes | Cook time: 55 minutes | Serves 8

1 teaspoon extra-virgin olive oil
1 sweet onion, chopped
1 tablespoon minced garlic
4 celery stalks, with the greens, chopped
3 carrots, peeled and diced
3 cups red lentils,
picked over, washed, and drained
4 cups low-sodium vegetable broth
3 cups water
2 bay leaves
2 teaspoons chopped fresh thyme
Sea salt and freshly ground black pepper, to taste

1. Place a large stockpot on medium-high heat and add the oil.
2. Sauté the onion and garlic until translucent, about 3 minutes.
3. Stir in the celery and carrots and sauté 5 minutes.
4. Add the lentils, broth, water, and bay leaves, and bring the soup to a boil.
5. Reduce the heat to low and simmer until the lentils are soft and the soup is thick, about 45 minutes.
6. Remove the bay leaves and stir in the thyme.
7. Season with salt and pepper and serve.

Per Serving
calories: 284 | fat:2 g | protein: 20g | carbs: 47g | sugars: 4g | fiber: 24g | sodium: 419mg

Turkey Cabbage Soup

Prep time: 15 minutes | Cook time: 30 minutes | Serves 4

1 tablespoon extra-virgin olive oil
1 sweet onion, chopped
2 celery stalks, chopped
2 teaspoons minced fresh garlic
4 cups finely shredded green cabbage
1 sweet potato,
peeled, diced
8 cups chicken or turkey broth
2 bay leaves
1 cup chopped cooked turkey
2 teaspoons chopped fresh thyme
Sea salt and freshly ground black pepper, to taste

1. Place a large saucepan over medium-high heat and add the olive oil.

2. Sauté the onion, celery, and garlic until softened and translucent, about 3 minutes.
3. Add the cabbage and sweet potato and sauté for 3 minutes.
4. Stir in the chicken broth and bay leaves and bring the soup to a boil.
5. Reduce the heat to low and simmer until the vegetables are tender, about 20 minutes.
6. Add the turkey and thyme and simmer until the turkey is heated through, about 4 minutes.
7. Remove the bay leaves and season the soup with salt and pepper.

Per Serving
calories: 325 | fat: 11g | protein: 24g | carbs: 30g | sugars: 13g | fiber: 4g | sodium: 715mg

Potlikker Soup

Prep time: 15 minutes | Cook time: 20 minutes | Serves 6

3 cups chicken broth, divided
1 medium onion, chopped
3 garlic cloves, minced
1 bunch collard greens or mustard greens including
stems, roughly chopped
1 fresh ham bone
5 carrots, peeled and cut into 1-inch rounds
2 fresh thyme sprigs
3 bay leaves
Freshly ground black pepper, to taste

1. Select the Sauté setting on an electric pressure cooker, and combine ½ cup of chicken broth, the onion, and garlic and cook for 3 to 5 minutes, or until the onion and garlic are translucent.
2. Add the collard greens, ham bone, carrots, remaining 2½ cups of broth, the thyme, and bay leaves.
3. Close and lock the lid and set the pressure valve to sealing.
4. Change to the Manual setting, and cook for 15 minutes.
5. Once cooking is complete, quick-release the pressure. Carefully remove the lid. Discard the bay leaves.
6. Serve with Skillet Bivalves.

Per Serving
calories: 99 | fat: 4g | protein: 6g | carbs: 10g | sugars: 4g | fiber: 3g | sodium: 201mg

Down South Corn Soup

Prep time: 10 minutes | Cook time: 35 minutes | Serves 8 to 10

1 tablespoon extra-virgin olive oil
½ Vidalia onion, minced
2 garlic cloves, minced
3 cups chopped cabbage
1 small cauliflower, broken into florets or 1 (10-ounce / 283-g) bag frozen cauliflower
1 (10-ounce / 283-g) bag frozen corn
1 cup vegetable broth
1 teaspoon smoked paprika
1 teaspoon ground cumin
1 teaspoon dried dill
½ teaspoon freshly ground black pepper
1 cup plain unsweetened cashew milk

1. In a large stockpot, heat the oil over medium heat.
2. Add the onion and garlic, and sauté, stirring to prevent the garlic from scorching, for 3 to 5 minutes, or until translucent.
3. Add the cabbage and a splash of water, cover, and cook for 5 minutes, or until tender.
4. Add the cauliflower, corn, broth, paprika, cumin, dill, and pepper. Cover and cook for 20 minutes, or until tender.
5. Add the cashew milk and stir well. Cover and cook for 5 minutes, letting the flavors come together.
6. Serve with a heaping plate of greens and seafood of your choice.

Per Serving
calories: 120 | fat: 4g | protein: 3g | carbs: 18g | sugars: 4g | fiber: 3g | sodium: 53mg

Carrot Soup

Prep time: 15 minutes | Cook time: 25 minutes | Serves 6

4 cups vegetable broth, divided
2 celery stalks, halved
1 small yellow onion, roughly chopped
½ fennel bulb, cored and roughly chopped
1 (1-inch) piece fresh ginger, peeled and chopped
1 pound (454 g) carrots, peeled and halved
2 teaspoons ground cumin
1 garlic clove, peeled
1 tablespoon almond butter

1. Select the Sauté setting on an electric pressure cooker, and combine ½ cup of broth, the celery, onion, fennel, and ginger. Cook for 5 minutes, or until the vegetables are tender.
2. Add the carrots, cumin, garlic, remaining 3½ cups of broth, and the almond butter.
3. Close and lock the lid, and set the pressure valve to sealing.
4. Change to the Manual setting, and cook for 15 minutes.
5. Once cooking is complete, quick-release the pressure. Carefully remove the lid, and let cool for 5 minutes.
6. Using a stand mixer or an immersion blender, carefully purée the soup. Serve with a heaping plate of greens.

Per Serving
calories: 82 | fat: 2g | protein: 3g | carbs: 13g | sugars: 5g | fiber: 3g | sodium: 121mg

Pumpkin Soup

Prep time: 15 minutes | Cook time: 30 minutes | Serves 6

2 cups seafood broth, divided
1 bunch collard greens, stemmed and cut into ribbons
1 tomato, chopped
1 garlic clove, minced
1 butternut squash or other winter squash,
peeled and cut into 1-inch cubes
1 teaspoon paprika
1 teaspoon dried dill
2 (5-ounce / 142-g) cans boneless, skinless salmon in water, rinsed

1. In a heavy-bottomed large stockpot, bring ½ cup of broth to a simmer over medium heat.
2. Add the collard greens, tomato, and garlic and cook for 5 minutes, or until the greens are wilted and the garlic is softened.
3. Add the squash, paprika, dill, and remaining 1½ cups of broth. Cover and cook for 20 minutes, or until the squash is tender.
4. Add the salmon and cook for 3 minutes, or just enough for the flavors to come together.

Per Serving
calories: 152 | fat: 2g | protein: 14g | carbs: 19g | sugars: 4g | fiber: 4g | sodium: 213mg

Beef Barley Soup

Prep time: 20 minutes | Cook time: 30 minutes | Serves 4

2 teaspoons extra-virgin olive oil
1 sweet onion, chopped
1 tablespoon minced garlic
4 celery stalks, with greens, chopped
2 carrots, peeled, diced
1 sweet potato, peeled, diced
8 cups low-sodium beef broth
1 cup cooked pearl barley
2 cups diced cooked beef
2 bay leaves
2 teaspoons hot sauce
2 teaspoons chopped fresh thyme
1 cup shredded kale
Sea salt and freshly ground black pepper, to taste

1. Place a large stockpot over medium-high heat and add the oil.
2. Sauté the onion and garlic until softened and translucent, about 3 minutes.
3. Stir in the celery, carrot, and sweet potato, and sauté for a further 5 minutes.
4. Stir in the beef broth, barley, beef, bay leaves, and hot sauce.
5. Bring the soup to a boil, then reduce the heat to low.
6. Simmer until the vegetables are tender, about 15 minutes.
7. Remove the bay leaves and stir in the thyme and kale.
8. Simmer for 5 minutes, and season with salt and pepper.

Per Serving
calories: 345 | fat: 11g | protein: 28g | carbs: 33g | sugars: 8g | fiber: 5g | sodium: 837mg

Seafood Stew

Prep time: 20 minutes | Cook time: 30 minutes | Serves 6

1 tablespoon extra-virgin olive oil
1 sweet onion, chopped
2 teaspoons minced garlic
3 celery stalks, chopped
2 carrots, peeled and chopped
1 (28-ounce / 794-g) can sodium-free diced tomatoes, undrained
3 cups low-sodium chicken broth
½ cup clam juice
¼ cup dry white wine
2 teaspoons chopped
fresh basil
2 teaspoons chopped fresh oregano
2 (4-ounce / 113-g) haddock fillets, cut into 1-inch chunks
1 pound (454 g) mussels, scrubbed, debearded
8 ounces (227 g) shrimp, peeled, deveined, quartered
Sea salt and freshly ground black pepper, to taste
2 tablespoons chopped fresh parsley

1. Place a large saucepan over medium-high heat and add the olive oil.
2. Sauté the onion and garlic until softened and translucent, about 3 minutes.
3. Stir in the celery and carrots and sauté for 4 minutes.
4. Stir in the tomatoes, chicken broth, clam juice, white wine, basil, and oregano.
5. Bring the sauce to a boil, then reduce the heat to low. Simmer for 15 minutes.
6. Add the fish and mussels, cover, and cook until the mussels open, about 5 minutes.
7. Discard any unopened mussels. Add the shrimp to the pan and cook until the shrimp are opaque, about 2 minutes.
8. Season with salt and pepper. Serve garnished with the chopped parsley.

Per Serving
calories: 248 | fat: 7g | protein: 28g | carbs: 19g | sugars: 7g | fiber: 2g | sodium: 577mg

Beef Barley Mushroom Soup

Prep time: 10 minutes | Cook time: 1 hour 20 minutes | Serves 6

1 pound (454 g) beef stew meat, cubed
¼ teaspoon salt
¼ teaspoon freshly ground black pepper
1 tablespoon extra-virgin olive oil
8 ounces (227 g) sliced mushrooms
1 onion, chopped
2 carrots, chopped
3 celery stalks, chopped
6 garlic cloves, minced
½ teaspoon dried thyme
4 cups low-sodium beef broth
1 cup water
½ cup pearl barley

1. Season the meat with the salt and pepper.
2. In an Instant Pot, heat the oil over high heat. Add the meat and brown on all sides. Remove the meat from the pot and set aside.
3. Add the mushrooms to the pot and cook for 1 to 2 minutes, until they begin to soften. Remove the mushrooms and set aside with the meat.
4. Add the onion, carrots, and celery to the pot. Sauté for 3 to 4 minutes until the vegetables begin to soften. Add the garlic and continue to cook until fragrant, about 30 seconds longer.
5. Return the meat and mushrooms to the pot, then add the thyme, beef broth, and water. Set the pressure to high and cook for 15 minutes. Let the pressure release naturally.
6. Open the Instant Pot and add the barley. Use the slow cooker function on the Instant Pot, affix the lid (vent open), and continue to cook for 1 hour until the barley is cooked through and tender. Serve.

Per Serving
calories: 246 | fat: 9g | protein: 21g | carbs: 19g | sugars: 3g | fiber: 4g | sodium: 516mg

White Bean and Butternut Squash Stew

Prep time: 16 minutes | Cook time: 7 minutes | Serves 6

1 pound (454 g) butternut squash, peeled, seeded, and cut into 1-inch cubes (about 3 cups)
1 tablespoon extra-virgin olive oil
1 tablespoon chili powder
1 teaspoon dried oregano
1 teaspoon ground cumin
1 tablespoon garlic pepper or garlic powder
½ teaspoon kosher salt
2 tablespoons finely chopped poblano chile or green bell pepper
3 cups vegetable broth or water
1 (15-ounce / 425-g) can diced tomatoes
1 (15-ounce / 425-g) can white beans, rinsed and drained
1 avocado, chopped just before serving

1. In the electric pressure cooker, toss the squash with the olive oil, chili powder, oregano, cumin, garlic pepper, and salt.
2. Stir in the poblano, broth, and tomatoes and their juices.
3. Close and lock the lid of the pressure cooker. Set the valve to sealing.
4. Cook on high pressure for 7 minutes.
5. When the cooking is complete, hit Cancel and quick release the pressure.
6. Once the pin drops, unlock and remove the lid.
7. Stir in the beans and let the stew sit for about 5 minutes to let the beans warm up.
8. Use an immersion blender to purée about one-third of the stew right in the pot. (I like to leave some chunks of squash and whole beans for more texture.)
9. Spoon into serving bowls and top with the avocado.

Per Serving (1 cup)
calories: 196 | fat: 6g | protein: 7g | carbs: 31g | sugars: 4g | fiber: 8g | sodium: 332mg

Buttercup Squash Soup

Prep time: 15 minutes | Cook time: 10 minutes | Serves 6

2 tablespoons extra-virgin olive oil
1 medium onion, chopped
4 to 5 cups vegetable broth or chicken bone broth
1½ pounds (680 g) buttercup squash, peeled, seeded, and cut into 1-inch chunks
½ teaspoon kosher salt
¼ teaspoon ground white pepper
Whole nutmeg, for grating

1. Set the electric pressure cooker to the Sauté setting. When the pot is hot, pour in the olive oil.
2. Add the onion and sauté for 3 to 5 minutes, until it begins to soften. Hit Cancel.
3. Add the broth, squash, salt, and pepper to the pot and stir. (If you want a thicker soup, use 4 cups of broth. If you want a thinner, drinkable soup, use 5 cups.)
4. Close and lock the lid of the pressure cooker. Set the valve to sealing.
5. Cook on high pressure for 10 minutes.
6. When the cooking is complete, hit Cancel and allow the pressure to release naturally.
7. Once the pin drops, unlock and remove the lid.
8. Use an immersion blender to purée the soup right in the pot. If you don't have an immersion blender, transfer the soup to a blender or food processor and purée. (Follow the instructions that came with your machine for blending hot foods.)
9. Pour the soup into serving bowls and grate nutmeg on top.

Per Serving (1¹/₃ cups)
calories: 111 | fat: 5g | protein:11 g | carbs: 18g | sugars: 4g | fiber: 4g | sodium: 166mg

Creamy Sweet Potato Soup

Prep time: 15 minutes | Cook time: 10 minutes | Serves 6

2 tablespoons avocado oil
1 small onion, chopped
2 celery stalks, chopped
2 teaspoons minced garlic
1 teaspoon kosher salt
½ teaspoon freshly ground black pepper
1 teaspoon ground turmeric
½ teaspoon ground cinnamon
2 pounds (907 g) sweet potatoes, peeled and cut into 1-inch cubes
3 cups vegetable broth or chicken bone broth
Plain Greek yogurt, to garnish (optional)
Chopped fresh parsley, to garnish (optional)
Pumpkin seeds (pepitas), to garnish (optional)

1. Set the electric pressure cooker to the Sauté setting. When the pot is hot, pour in the avocado oil.
2. Sauté the onion and celery for 3 to 5 minutes or until the vegetables begin to soften.
3. Stir in the garlic, salt, pepper, turmeric, and cinnamon. Hit Cancel.
4. Stir in the sweet potatoes and broth.
5. Close and lock the lid of the pressure cooker. Set the valve to sealing.
6. Cook on high pressure for 10 minutes.
7. When the cooking is complete, hit Cancel and allow the pressure to release naturally.
8. Once the pin drops, unlock and remove the lid.
9. Use an immersion blender to purée the soup right in the pot. If you don't have an immersion blender, transfer the soup to a blender or food processor and purée. (Follow the instructions that came with your machine for blending hot foods.)
10. Spoon into bowls and serve topped with Greek yogurt, parsley, and/or pumpkin seeds (if using).

Per Serving (1 cup)
calories: 193 | fat: 5g | protein: 3g | carbs: 36g | sugars: 8g | fiber: 6g | sodium: 302mg

Bean Soup with Lime-Yogurt Drizzle

Prep time: 10 minutes | Cook time: 40 minutes | Serves 8

2 tablespoons avocado oil
1 medium onion, chopped
3 garlic cloves, minced
1 teaspoon ground cumin
1 (10-ounce / 283-g) can diced tomatoes and green chilies
6 cups chicken bone broth, vegetable broth, or water
1 pound (454 g) dried black beans, rinsed
Kosher salt, to taste
¼ cup plain Greek yogurt or sour cream
1 tablespoon freshly squeezed lime juice

1. Set the electric pressure cooker to the Sauté setting. When the pot is hot, pour in the avocado oil.
2. Sauté the onion for 3 to 5 minutes, until it begins to soften. Hit Cancel.
3. Stir in the garlic, cumin, tomatoes and their juices, broth, and beans.
4. Close and lock the lid of the pressure cooker. Set the valve to sealing.
5. Cook on high pressure for 40 minutes.
6. While the soup is cooking, combine the yogurt and lime juice in a small bowl.
7. When the cooking is complete, hit Cancel. Allow the pressure to release naturally for 15 minutes, then quick release any remaining pressure.
8. Once the pin drops, unlock and remove the lid.
9. (Optional) For a thicker soup, remove 1½ cups of beans from the pot using a slotted spoon. Use an immersion blender to blend the beans that remain in the pot. If you don't have an immersion blender, transfer the soup left in the pot to a blender or food processor and purée. (Follow the instructions that came with your machine for blending hot foods.) Stir in the reserved beans. Season with salt, if desired.
10. Spoon into serving bowls and drizzle with lime-yogurt sauce.

Per Serving (1 cup)
calories: 285 | fat: 6g | protein: 19g | carbs: 42g | sugars: 3g | fiber: 10g | sodium: 174mg

Chicken Noodle Soup

Prep time: 15 minutes | Cook time: 20 minutes | Serves 12

2 tablespoons avocado oil
1 medium onion, chopped
3 celery stalks, chopped
1 teaspoon kosher salt
¼ teaspoon freshly ground black pepper
2 teaspoons minced garlic
5 large carrots, peeled and cut into ¼-inch-thick rounds
3 pounds (1.4 kg) bone-in chicken breasts (about 3)
4 cups chicken bone broth
4 cups water
2 tablespoons soy sauce
6 ounces (170 g) whole grain wide egg noodles

1. Set the electric pressure cooker to the Sauté setting. When the pot is hot, pour in the avocado oil.
2. Sauté the onion, celery, salt, and pepper for 3 to 5 minutes or until the vegetables begin to soften.
3. Add the garlic and carrots, and stir to mix well. Hit Cancel.
4. Add the chicken to the pot, meat-side down. Add the broth, water, and soy sauce. Close and lock the lid of the pressure cooker. Set the valve to sealing.
5. Cook on high pressure for 20 minutes.
6. When the cooking is complete, hit Cancel and quick release the pressure. Unlock and remove the lid.
7. Using tongs, remove the chicken breasts to a cutting board. Hit Sauté/More and bring the soup to a boil.
8. Add the noodles and cook for 4 to 5 minutes or until the noodles are al dente.
9. While the noodles are cooking, use two forks to shred the chicken. Add the meat back to the pot and save the bones to make more bone broth.
10. Season with additional pepper, if desired, and serve.

Per Serving (1 cup)
calories: 330 | fat: 15g | protein: 32g | carbs: 17g | sugars: 3g | fiber: 4g | sodium: 451mg

Turkey Barley Vegetable Soup

Prep time: 5 minutes | Cook time: 20 minutes | Serves 8

2 tablespoons avocado oil
1 pound (454 g) ground turkey
4 cups chicken bone broth, low-sodium store-bought chicken broth, or water
1 (28-ounce / 794-g) carton or can diced tomatoes
2 tablespoons tomato paste
1 (15-ounce / 425-g) package frozen chopped carrots (about 2½ cups)
1 (15-ounce / 425-g) package frozen peppers and onions (about 2½ cups)
⅓ cup dry barley
1 teaspoon kosher salt
¼ teaspoon freshly ground black pepper
2 bay leaves

1. Set the electric pressure cooker to the Sauté/More setting. When the pot is hot, pour in the avocado oil.
2. Add the turkey to the pot and sauté, stirring frequently to break up the meat, for about 7 minutes or until the turkey is no longer pink. Hit Cancel.
3. Add the broth, tomatoes and their juices, and tomato paste. Stir in the carrots, peppers and onions, barley, salt, pepper, and bay leaves.
4. Close and lock the lid of the pressure cooker. Set the valve to sealing.
5. Cook on high pressure for 20 minutes.
6. When the cooking is complete, hit Cancel and allow the pressure to release naturally for 10 minutes, then quick release any remaining pressure.
7. Once the pin drops, unlock and remove the lid. Discard the bay leaves.
8. Spoon into bowls and serve.

Per Serving (1¼ cups)
calories: 253 | fat: 12g | protein: 19g | carbs:21 g | sugars: 7g | fiber: 7g | sodium: 560mg

Minestrone with Red Beans and Zucchini

Prep time: 15 minutes | Cook time: 5 minutes | Serves 8

Soup:
2 tablespoons avocado oil
1 cup chopped onion
1 celery stalk, chopped
1 teaspoon dried thyme
½ teaspoon dried sage leaves
½ teaspoon freshly ground black pepper
2 cups vegetable broth or water
1 (28-ounce / 794-g) carton or can chopped tomatoes
1 (15-ounce / 425-g) can small red beans, rinsed and drained
2 carrots, peeled and chopped
2 bay leaves
½ cup whole wheat orzo, uncooked (optional)

Finish:
1 medium zucchini, quartered lengthwise, then chopped
2 cups baby spinach
¼ cup freshly grated Parmesan cheese
Chopped fresh basil (optional)

Make the Soup
1. Set the electric pressure cooker to the Sauté setting. When the pot is hot, pour in the avocado oil.
2. Sauté the onion and celery for 3 to 5 minutes, or until the vegetables begin to soften. Stir in the thyme, sage, and pepper. Hit Cancel.
3. Add the broth, tomatoes and their juices, beans, carrots, bay leaves, and orzo (if using).
4. Close and lock the lid of the pressure cooker. Set the valve to sealing.
5. Cook on high pressure for 5 minutes.
6. When the cooking is complete, hit Cancel and quick release the pressure.
7. Once the pin drops, unlock and remove the lid.

Finish the Soup
1. Stir in the zucchini and spinach. Replace the lid and let the pot sit for 10 minutes.
2. Spoon into serving bowls and top with the Parmesan cheese and basil (if using).

Per Serving (1 cup)
calories: 152 | fat: 5g | protein: 6g | carbs: 23g | sugars: 8g | fiber: 7g | sodium: 357mg

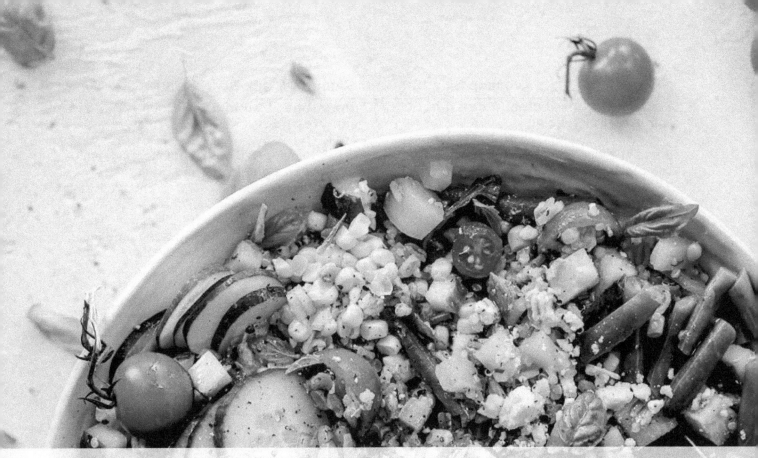

Chapter 4 Salads, Sides, and Snacks

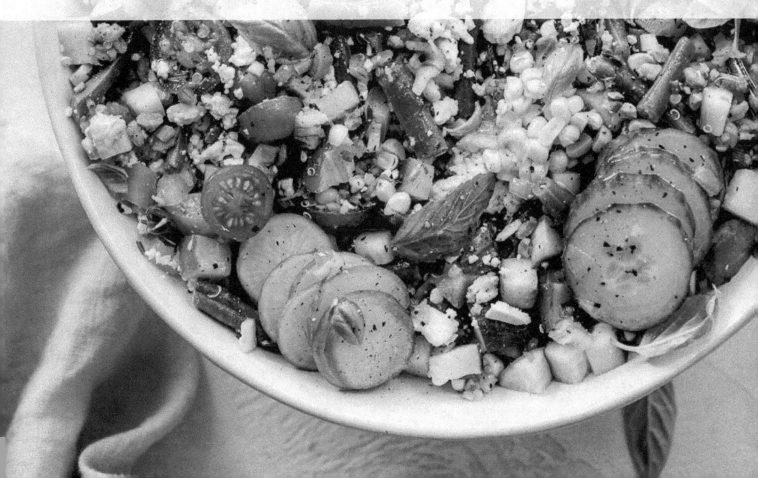

Cucumber Tomato Avocado Salad

Prep time: 10 minutes | Cook time: 0 minutes | Serves 4

1 cup cherry tomatoes, halved
1 large cucumber, chopped
1 small red onion, thinly sliced
1 avocado, diced
2 tablespoons

chopped fresh dill
2 tablespoons extra-virgin olive oil
Juice of 1 lemon
¼ teaspoon salt
¼ teaspoon freshly ground black pepper

1. In a large mixing bowl, combine the tomatoes, cucumber, onion, avocado, and dill.
2. In a small bowl, combine the oil, lemon juice, salt, and pepper, and mix well.
3. Drizzle the dressing over the vegetables and toss to combine. Serve.

Per Serving

calories: 151 | fat: 12g | protein: 2g | carbs: 11g | sugars: 4g | fiber: 4g | sodium: 128mg

Garlicky Cabbage and Collard Greens

Prep time: 10 minutes | Cook time: 10 minutes | Serves 8

2 tablespoons extra-virgin olive oil
1 collard greens bunch, stemmed and thinly sliced
½ small green

cabbage, thinly sliced
6 garlic cloves, minced
1 tablespoon low-sodium gluten-free soy sauce or tamari

1. In a large skillet, heat the oil over medium-high heat.
2. Add the collards to the pan, stirring to coat with oil. Sauté for 1 to 2 minutes until the greens begin to wilt.
3. Add the cabbage and stir to coat. Cover and reduce the heat to medium low. Continue to cook for 5 to 7 minutes, stirring once or twice, until the greens are tender.
4. Add the garlic and soy sauce and stir to incorporate. Cook until just fragrant, about 30 seconds longer. Serve warm and enjoy!

Per Serving

calories: 72 | fat: 4g | protein: 3g | carbs: 6g | sugars: 0g | fiber: 3g | sodium: 129mg

Rainbow Black Bean Salad

Prep time: 15 minutes | Cook time: 0 minutes | Serves 5

1 (15-ounce / 425-g) can low-sodium black beans, drained and rinsed
1 avocado, diced
1 cup cherry tomatoes, halved
1 cup chopped baby spinach
½ cup finely chopped red bell pepper
¼ cup finely chopped jicama
½ cup chopped

scallions, both white and green parts
¼ cup chopped fresh cilantro
2 tablespoons freshly squeezed lime juice
1 tablespoon extra-virgin olive oil
2 garlic cloves, minced
1 teaspoon honey
¼ teaspoon salt
¼ teaspoon freshly ground black pepper

1. In a large bowl, combine the black beans, avocado, tomatoes, spinach, bell pepper, jicama, scallions, and cilantro.
2. In a small bowl, mix the lime juice, oil, garlic, honey, salt, and pepper. Add to the salad and toss.
3. Chill for 1 hour before serving.

Per Serving

calories: 169 | fat: 7g | protein: 6g | carbs: 22g | sugars: 3g | fiber: 9g | sodium: 235mg

Veggies with Cottage Cheese Ranch Dip

Prep time: 10 minutes | Cook time: 0 minutes | Serves 4

1 cup cottage cheese
2 tablespoons mayonnaise
Juice of ½ lemon
2 tablespoons chopped fresh chives
2 tablespoons chopped fresh dill

2 scallions, white and green parts, finely chopped
1 garlic clove, minced
½ teaspoon sea salt
2 zucchinis, cut into sticks
8 cherry tomatoes

1. In a small bowl, mix the cottage cheese, mayonnaise, lemon juice, chives, dill, scallions, garlic, and salt.
2. Serve with the zucchini sticks and cherry tomatoes for dipping.

Per Serving

calories: 90 | fat: 4g | protein: 7g | carbs: 7g | sugars: 5g | fiber: 1g | sodium: 387mg

Cinnamon Toasted Pumpkin Seeds

Prep time: 5 minutes | Cook time: 45 minutes | Serves 4

1 cup pumpkin seeds
2 tablespoons canola oil
1 teaspoon cinnamon
2 (1-gram) packets stevia
¼ teaspoon sea salt

1. Preheat the oven to 300ºF (150ºC).
2. In a bowl, toss the pumpkin seeds with the oil, cinnamon, stevia, and salt.
3. Spread the seeds in a single layer on a rimmed baking sheet. Bake until browned and fragrant, stirring once or twice, about 45 minutes.

Per Serving

calories: 135 | fat: 10g | protein: 3g | carbs: 9g | sugars: 0g | fiber: 1g | sodium: 76mg

Garlic and Basil Three Bean Salad

Prep time: 10 minutes | Cook time: 0 minutes | Serves 8

1 (15-ounce / 425-g) can low-sodium chickpeas, drained and rinsed
1 (15-ounce / 425-g) can low-sodium kidney beans, drained and rinsed
1 (15-ounce / 425-g) can low-sodium white beans, drained and rinsed
1 red bell pepper, seeded and finely chopped
¼ cup chopped scallions, both white and green parts
¼ cup finely chopped fresh basil
3 garlic cloves, minced
2 tablespoons extra-virgin olive oil
1 tablespoon red wine vinegar
1 teaspoon Dijon mustard
¼ teaspoon freshly ground black pepper

1. In a large mixing bowl, combine the chickpeas, kidney beans, white beans, bell pepper, scallions, basil, and garlic. Toss gently to combine.
2. In a small bowl, combine the olive oil, vinegar, mustard, and pepper. Toss with the salad.
3. Cover and refrigerate for an hour before serving, to allow the flavors to mix.

Per Serving

calories: 193 | fat: 5g | protein: 10g | carbs: 29g | sugars: 3g | fiber: 8g | sodium: 246mg

Cocoa Coated Almonds

Prep time: 5 minutes | Cook time: 15 minutes | Serves 4

1 cup almonds
1 tablespoon cocoa powder
2 packets powdered stevia

1. Preheat the oven to 350ºF (180ºC). Line a baking sheet with parchment paper.
2. Spread the almonds in a single layer on the baking sheet. Bake for 5 minutes.
3. While the almonds bake, in a small bowl, mix the cocoa and stevia well. Add the hot almonds to the bowl. Toss to combine.
4. Return the almonds to the baking sheet and bake until fragrant, about 5 minutes more.

Per Serving

calories: 209 | fat: 1g | protein: 8g | carbs: 9g | sugars: 1g | fiber: 5g | sodium: 1mg

Blueberry Chicken Salad

Prep time: 10 minutes | Cook time: 0 minutes | Serves 4

2 cups chopped cooked chicken
1 cup fresh blueberries
¼ cup finely chopped almonds
1 celery stalk, finely chopped
¼ cup finely chopped red onion
1 tablespoon chopped fresh basil
1 tablespoon chopped fresh cilantro
½ cup plain, nonfat Greek yogurt or vegan mayonnaise
¼ teaspoon salt
¼ teaspoon freshly ground black pepper
8 cups salad greens (baby spinach, spicy greens, romaine)

1. In a large mixing bowl, combine the chicken, blueberries, almonds, celery, onion, basil, and cilantro. Toss gently to mix.
2. In a small bowl, combine the yogurt, salt, and pepper. Add to the chicken salad and stir to combine.
3. Arrange 2 cups of salad greens on each of 4 plates and divide the chicken salad among the plates to serve.

Per Serving

calories: 207 | fat: 6g | protein: 28g | carbs: 11g | sugars: 6g | fiber: 3g | sodium: 235mg

Roasted Delicata Squash

Prep time: 10 minutes | Cook time: 20 minutes | Serves 4

1 (1- to 1½-pound / 454- to 680-g) delicata squash, halved, seeded, cut into ½-inch-thick strips
1 tablespoon extra-

virgin olive oil
½ teaspoon dried thyme
¼ teaspoon salt
¼ teaspoon freshly ground black pepper

1. Preheat the oven to 400ºF (205ºC). Line a baking sheet with parchment paper.
2. In a large mixing bowl, toss the squash strips with the olive oil, thyme, salt, and pepper. Arrange on the prepared baking sheet in a single layer.
3. Roast for 10 minutes, flip, and continue to roast for 10 more minutes until tender and lightly browned.

Per Serving
calories: 79 | fat: 4g | protein: 1g | carbs: 12g | sugars: 3g | fiber: 2g | sodium: 123mg

Roasted Asparagus, Onions, and Red Peppers

Prep time: 5 minutes | Cook time: 20 minutes | Serves 4

1 pound (454 g) asparagus, woody ends trimmed, cut into 2-inch segments
1 small onion, quartered

2 red bell peppers, seeded, cut into 1-inch pieces
2 tablespoons Easy Italian Dressing (see recipe)

1. Preheat the oven to 400ºF (205ºC). Line a baking sheet with parchment paper.
2. In a large mixing bowl, toss the asparagus, onion, and peppers with the dressing. Transfer to the prepared baking sheet.
3. Roast for 10 minutes, then, using a spatula, flip the vegetables. Roast for 5 to 10 more minutes until the vegetables are tender.
4. Stir well and serve.

Per Serving
calories: 93 | fat: 5g | protein: 3g | carbs: 11g | sugars: 6g | fiber: 4g | sodium: 32mg

Tomato, Peach, and Strawberry Salad

Prep time: 15 minutes | Cook time: 0 minutes | Serves 6

6 cups mixed spring greens
4 large ripe plum tomatoes, thinly sliced
4 large ripe peaches, pitted and thinly sliced
12 ripe strawberries,

thinly sliced
½ Vidalia onion, thinly sliced
2 tablespoons white balsamic vinegar
2 tablespoons extra-virgin olive oil
Freshly ground black pepper, to taste

1. Put the greens in a large salad bowl, and layer the tomatoes, peaches, strawberries, and onion on top.
2. Dress with the vinegar and oil, toss together, and season with pepper.

Per Serving
calories: 127 | fat: 5g | protein: 4g | carbs: 19g | sugars: 13g | fiber: 5g | sodium: 30mg

Raw Corn Salad with Black-Eyed Peas

Prep time: 15 minutes | Cook time: 0 minutes | Serves 8

2 ears fresh corn, kernels cut off
2 cups cooked black-eyed peas
1 green bell pepper, chopped
½ red onion, chopped
2 celery stalks, finely chopped
½ pint cherry tomatoes, halved

3 tablespoons white balsamic vinegar
2 tablespoons extra-virgin olive oil
1 garlic clove, minced
¼ teaspoon smoked paprika
¼ teaspoon ground cumin
¼ teaspoon red pepper flakes

1. In a large salad bowl, combine the corn, black-eyed peas, bell pepper, onion, celery, and tomatoes.
2. In a small bowl, to make the dressing, whisk the vinegar, olive oil, garlic, paprika, cumin, and red pepper flakes together.
3. Pour the dressing over the salad, and toss gently to coat. Serve and enjoy.

Per Serving
calories: 123 | fat: 5g | protein: 5g | carbs: 18g | sugars: 3g | fiber: 4g | sodium: 24mg

Peanut Butter Protein Bites

Prep time: 10 minutes | Cook time: 0 minutes | Makes 16 balls

½ cup sugar-free peanut butter
¼ cup (1 scoop) sugar-free peanut butter powder or sugar-free protein powder

2 tablespoons unsweetened cocoa powder
2 tablespoons canned coconut milk (or more to adjust consistency)

1. In a bowl, mix all ingredients until well combined.
2. Roll into 16 balls. Refrigerate before serving.

Per Serving (1 ball)
calories: 61 | fat: 5g | protein: 4g | carbs: 2g | sugars: 2g | fiber: 0g | sodium: 19mg

Spaghetti Squash

Prep time: 5 minutes | Cook time: 7 minutes | Serves 4

1 spaghetti squash (about 2 pounds / 907 g)

1. Cut the spaghetti squash in half crosswise and use a large spoon to remove the seeds.
2. Pour 1 cup of water into the electric pressure cooker and insert a wire rack or trivet.
3. Place the squash halves on the rack, cut-side up.
4. Close and lock the lid of the pressure cooker. Set the valve to sealing.
5. Cook on high pressure for 7 minutes.
6. When the cooking is complete, hit Cancel and quick release the pressure.
7. Once the pin drops, unlock and remove the lid.
8. With tongs, remove the squash from the pot and transfer it to a plate. When it is cool enough to handle, scrape the squash with the tines of a fork to remove the strands. Discard the skin.

Per Serving
calories: 10 | fat: 0g | protein: 0g | carbs: 3g | sugars: 1g | fiber: 1g | sodium: 17mg

Almond Milk Nut Butter Mocha Smoothie

Prep time: 5 minutes | Cook time: 0 minutes | Serves 1

1 cup almond milk
2 tablespoons almond butter
1 tablespoon cocoa powder
1 teaspoon espresso powder (or to taste)

1 to 2 (1-gram) packets stevia (or to taste)
¼ teaspoon almond extract
½ cup crushed ice

1. In a blender, combine all of the ingredients and blend on high until smooth.

Per Serving
calories: 242 | fat: 21g | protein: 10g | carbs: 12g | sugars: 12g | fiber: 6g | sodium: 66mg

Candied Yams

Prep time: 7 minutes | Cook time: 45 minutes | Serves 8

2 medium jewel yams, cut into 2-inch dice
Juice of 1 large orange
2 tablespoons unsalted non-hydrogenated plant-based butter

1½ teaspoons ground cinnamon
¾ teaspoon ground nutmeg
¼ teaspoon ground ginger
⅛ teaspoon ground cloves

1. Preheat the oven to 350ºF (180ºC).
2. On a rimmed baking sheet, arrange the diced yam in a single layer.
3. In a medium pot, combine the orange juice, butter, cinnamon, nutmeg, ginger, and cloves and cook over medium-low heat for 3 to 5 minutes, or until the ingredients come together and thicken.
4. Pour the hot juice mixture over the yams, turning them to make sure they are evenly coated.
5. Transfer the baking sheet to the oven, and bake for 40 minutes, or until the yams are tender.

Per Serving
calories: 130 | fat: 3g | protein: 2g | carbs: 25g | sugars: 3g | fiber: 5g | sodium: 30mg

Young Kale and Cabbage Salad

Prep time: 15 minutes | Cook time: 0 minutes | Serves 6

2 bunches baby kale, thinly sliced
½ head green savoy cabbage, cored and thinly sliced
¼ cup apple cider vinegar
Juice of 1 lemon
1 teaspoon ground cumin
¼ teaspoon smoked paprika
1 medium red bell pepper, thinly sliced
1 cup toasted peanuts
1 garlic clove, thinly sliced

1. In a large salad bowl, toss the kale and cabbage together.
2. In a small bowl, to make the dressing, whisk the vinegar, lemon juice, cumin, and paprika together.
3. Pour the dressing over the greens, and gently massage with your hands.
4. Add the pepper, peanuts, and garlic, and toss to combine.

Per Serving
calories: 199 | fat: 12g | protein: 10g | carbs: 17g | sugars: 4g | fiber: 5g | sodium: 46mg

Spicy Roasted Cauliflower with Lime

Prep time: 5 minutes | Cook time: 10 minutes | Serves 4

1 cauliflower head, broken into small florets
2 tablespoons extra-virgin olive oil
½ teaspoon ground chipotle chili powder
½ teaspoon salt
Juice of 1 lime

1. Preheat the oven to 450°F (235°C). Line a rimmed baking sheet with parchment paper.
2. In a large mixing bowl, toss the cauliflower with the olive oil, chipotle chili powder, and salt. Arrange in a single layer on the prepared baking sheet.
3. Roast for 15 minutes, flip, and continue to roast for 15 more minutes until well-browned and tender.
4. Sprinkle with the lime juice, adjust the salt as needed, and serve.

Per Serving
calories: 99 | fat: 7g | protein: 3g | carbs: 8g | sugars: 3g | fiber: 3g | sodium: 284mg

Summer Salad

Prep time: 5 minutes | Cook time: 0 minutes | Serves 4

Salad:
8 cups mixed greens or preferred lettuce, loosely packed
4 cups arugula, loosely packed
2 peaches, sliced ½
cup thinly sliced red onion
½ cup chopped walnuts or pecans
½ cup crumbled feta
Dressing:
4 teaspoons extra-virgin olive oil
4 teaspoons honey

Make the Salad
1. Combine the mixed greens, arugula, peaches, red onion, walnuts, and feta in a large bowl. Divide the salad into four portions.
2. Drizzle the dressing over each individual serving of salad.

Make the Dressing
1. In a small bowl, whisk together the olive oil and honey.

Per Serving
calories: 263 | fat: 18g | protein: 8g | carbs: 22g | sugars: 16g | fiber: 5g | sodium: 222mg

Turkey Rollups with Veggie Cream Cheese

Prep time: 10 minutes | Cook time: 0 minutes | Serves 2

¼ cup cream cheese, at room temperature
2 tablespoons finely chopped red onion
2 tablespoons finely chopped red bell pepper
1 tablespoon chopped fresh chives
1 teaspoon Dijon mustard
1 garlic clove, minced
¼ teaspoon sea salt
6 slices deli turkey

1. In a small bowl, mix the cream cheese, red onion, bell pepper, chives, mustard, garlic, and salt.
2. Spread the mixture on the turkey slices and roll up.

Per Serving
calories: 146 | fat: 10g | protein: 8g | carbs: 5g | sugars: 6g | fiber: 1g | sodium: 914mg

Guacamole with Jicama

Prep time: 5 minutes | Cook time: 0 minutes | Serves 4

1 avocado, cut into cubes
Juice of ½ lime
2 tablespoons finely chopped red onion

2 tablespoons chopped fresh cilantro
1 garlic clove, minced
¼ teaspoon sea salt
1 cup sliced jicama

1. In a small bowl, combine the avocado, lime juice, onion, cilantro, garlic, and salt. Mash lightly with a fork.
2. Serve with the jicama for dipping.

Per Serving

calories: 73 | fat: 5g | protein: 1g | carbs: 8g | sugars: 1g | fiber: 5g | sodium: 77mg

Zucchini Hummus Dip with Red Peppers

Prep time: 10 minutes | Cook time: 0 minutes | Serves 4

2 zucchini, chopped
3 garlic cloves
2 tablespoons extra-virgin olive oil
2 tablespoons tahini

Juice of 1 lemon
½ teaspoon sea salt
1 red bell pepper, seeded and cut into sticks

1. In a blender or food processor, combine the zucchini, garlic, olive oil, tahini, lemon juice, and salt. Blend until smooth.
2. Serve with the red bell pepper for dipping.

Per Serving

calories: 121 | fat: 11g | protein: 2g | carbs: 7g | sugars: 1g | fiber: 3g | sodium: 156mg

Garlic Kale Chips

Prep time: 5 minutes | Cook time: 15 minutes | Serves 1

1 (8-ounce / 227-g) bunch kale, trimmed and cut into 2-inch pieces
1 tablespoon extra-virgin olive oil

½ teaspoon sea salt
¼ teaspoon garlic powder
Pinch cayenne (optional, to taste)

1. Preheat the oven to 350ºF (180ºC). Line two baking sheets with parchment paper.
2. Wash the kale and pat it completely dry.

3. In a large bowl, toss the kale with the olive oil, sea salt, garlic powder, and cayenne, if using.
4. Spread the kale in a single layer on the prepared baking sheets.
5. Bake until crisp, 12 to 15 minutes, rotating the sheets once.

Per Serving

calories: 231 | fat: 15g | protein: 7g | carbs: 20g | sugars: 0g | fiber: 4g | sodium: 678mg

Buffalo Chicken Celery Sticks

Prep time: 10 minutes | Cook time: 0 minutes | Serves 4

1 cup shredded cooked rotisserie chicken meat
¼ cup chunky blue cheese dressing

1 teaspoon Louisiana hot sauce
8 celery stalks, cut into halves lengthwise

1. In a small bowl, mix the chicken, blue cheese dressing, and hot sauce.
2. Spread the mixture into the celery stalks.

Per Serving

calories: 149 | fat: 12g | protein: 9g | carbs: 3g | sugars: 1g | fiber: 1g | sodium: 463mg

Baked Parmesan Crisps

Prep time: 5 minutes | Cook time: 5 minutes | Serves 2

1 cup grated Parmesan cheese

1. Preheat the oven to 400ºF (205ºC). Line a rimmed baking sheet with parchment paper.
2. Spread the Parmesan on the prepared baking sheet into 4 mounds, spreading each mound out so it is flat but not touching the others.
3. Bake until brown and crisp, 3 to 5 minutes.
4. Cool for 5 minutes. Use a spatula to remove to a plate to continue cooling.

Per Serving

calories: 216 | fat: 14g | protein: 19g | carbs: 2g | sugars: 0g | fiber: 0g | sodium: 765mg

Pear, Walnut, and Spinach Salad

Prep time: 10 minutes | Cook time: 0 minutes | Serves 2

4 cups baby spinach
½ pear, cored, peeled, and chopped
¼ cup whole walnuts, chopped
2 tablespoons apple cider vinegar
2 tablespoons extra-

virgin olive oil
1 teaspoon peeled and grated fresh ginger
½ teaspoon Dijon mustard
½ teaspoon sea salt

1. Layer the spinach on the bottom of two mason jars. Top with the pear and walnuts.
2. In a small bowl, whisk together the vinegar, oil, ginger, mustard, and salt. Put in another lidded container.
3. Shake the dressing before serving and add it to the mason jars. Close the jars and shake to distribute the dressing.

Per Serving
calories: 254 | fat: 23g | protein: 4g | carbs: 10g | sugars: 4g | fiber: 4g | sodium: 340mg

Winter Chicken Salad with Citrus

Prep time: 10 minutes | Cook time: 0 minutes | Serves 4

4 cups baby spinach
2 tablespoons extra-virgin olive oil
1 tablespoon freshly squeezed lemon juice
⅛ teaspoon salt
Freshly ground black pepper, to taste

2 cups chopped cooked chicken
2 mandarin oranges, peeled and sectioned
½ peeled grapefruit, sectioned
¼ cup sliced almonds

1. In a large mixing bowl, toss the spinach with the olive oil, lemon juice, salt, and pepper.
2. Add the chicken, oranges, grapefruit, and almonds to the bowl. Toss gently.
3. Arrange on 4 plates and serve.

Per Serving
calories: 249 | fat: 12g | protein: 24g | carbs: 11g | sugars: 7g | fiber: 3g | sodium: 135mg

Sautéed Spinach and Cherry Tomatoes

Prep time: 5 minutes | Cook time: 10 minutes | Serves 4

1 tablespoon extra-virgin olive oil
1 cup cherry tomatoes, halved
3 spinach bunches,

trimmed
2 garlic cloves, minced
¼ teaspoon salt

1. In a large skillet, heat the oil over medium heat.
2. Add the tomatoes, and cook until the skins begin to blister and split, about 2 minutes.
3. Add the spinach in batches, waiting for each batch to wilt slightly before adding the next batch. Stir continuously for 3 to 4 minutes until the spinach is tender.
4. Add the garlic to the skillet, and toss until fragrant, about 30 seconds.
5. Drain the excess liquid from the pan. Add the salt. Stir well and serve.

Per Serving
calories: 52 | fat: 4g | protein: 2g | carbs: 4g | sugars: 1g | fiber: 2g | sodium: 183mg

Roasted Lemon and Garlic Broccoli

Prep time: 10 minutes | Cook time: 25 minutes | Serves 8

2 large broccoli heads, cut into florets
3 garlic cloves, minced
2 tablespoons extra-virgin olive oil

¼ teaspoon salt
¼ teaspoon freshly ground black pepper
2 tablespoons freshly squeezed lemon juice

1. Preheat the oven to 425ºF (220ºC).
2. On a rimmed baking sheet, toss the broccoli, garlic, and olive oil. Season with the salt and pepper.
3. Roast, tossing occasionally, for 25 to 30 minutes until tender and browned. Season with the lemon juice and serve.

Per Serving
calories: 30 | fat: 2g | protein: 1g | carbs: 3g | sugars: 1g | fiber: 1g | sodium: 84mg

Cauli-Broccoli Tots

Prep time: 10 minutes | Cook time: 20 minutes | Serves 4

1 cup chopped broccoli florets and stems
1 cup chopped cauliflower florets and stems
¼ cup diced onion
1 large egg
¼ cup whole-wheat bread crumbs
¼ cup crumbled feta cheese
½ teaspoon salt
¼ teaspoon freshly ground black pepper

1. Preheat the oven to 400ºF (205ºC). Line a baking sheet with parchment paper.
2. In a food processor, combine the broccoli, cauliflower, and onion, and pulse until chopped well but still slightly chunky. Or if you don't have a food processor, chop everything on a large cutting board until you have very small pieces. Transfer to a large mixing bowl.
3. Add the egg, bread crumbs, cheese, salt, and pepper.
4. Using your hands, shape small balls, a little smaller than a tablespoon, and carefully place them on the prepared baking sheet.
5. Bake for 10 minutes, flip carefully, and continue to bake for 10 additional minutes until browned and crisp.

Per Serving
calories: 90 | fat: 4g | protein: 5g | carbs: 9g | sugars: 2g | fiber: 2g | sodium: 424mg

Blackberry Goat Cheese Salad

Prep time: 15 minutes | Cook time: 20 minutes | Serves 4

Vinaigrette:
1 pint blackberries
2 tablespoons red wine vinegar
1 tablespoon honey
3 tablespoons extra-
virgin olive oil
¼ teaspoon salt
Freshly ground black pepper, to taste
Salad:
1 sweet potato, cubed
1 teaspoon extra-virgin olive oil
8 cups salad greens (baby spinach, spicy
greens, romaine)
½ red onion, sliced
¼ cup crumbled goat cheese

Make the Vinaigrette
1. In a blender jar, combine the blackberries, vinegar, honey, oil, salt, and pepper, and process until smooth. Set aside.

Make the Salad
1. Preheat the oven to 425ºF (220ºC). Line a baking sheet with parchment paper.
2. In a medium mixing bowl, toss the sweet potato with the olive oil. Transfer to the prepared baking sheet and roast for 20 minutes, stirring once halfway through, until tender. Remove and cool for a few minutes.
3. In a large bowl, toss the greens with the red onion and cooled sweet potato, and drizzle with the vinaigrette. Serve topped with 1 tablespoon of goat cheese Per Serving.

Per Serving
calories: 196 | fat: 12g | protein: 3g | carbs: 21g | sugars: 10g | fiber: 6g | sodium: 184mg

Sofrito Steak Salad

Prep time: 10 minutes | Cook time: 15 minutes | Serves 4

4 ounces (113 g) recaíto cooking base
2 (4-ounce / 113-g) flank steaks
8 cups fresh spinach, loosely packed
½ cup sliced red
onion
2 cups diced tomato
2 avocados, diced
2 cups diced cucumber
⅓ cup crumbled feta

1. Heat a large skillet over medium-low heat. When hot, pour in the recaíto cooking base, add the steaks, and cover. Cook for 8 to 12 minutes.
2. Meanwhile, divide the spinach into four portions. Top each portion with one-quarter of the onion, tomato, avocados, and cucumber.
3. Remove the steak from the skillet, and let it rest for about 2 minutes before slicing. Place one-quarter of the steak and feta on top of each portion.

Per Serving
calories: 344 | fat: 18g | protein: 25g | carbs: 18g | sugars: 6g | fiber: 8g | sodium: 382mg

Chicken, Spinach, and Berry Salad

Prep time: 5 minutes | Cook time: 0 minutes | Serves 4

Salad:

8 cups baby spinach
2 cups shredded rotisserie chicken
½ cup sliced strawberries or other
berries
½ cup sliced almonds
1 avocado, sliced
¼ cup crumbled feta (optional)

Dressing:

2 tablespoons extra-virgin olive oil
2 teaspoons honey
2 teaspoons balsamic vinegar

Make the Salad

1. In a large bowl, combine the spinach, chicken, strawberries, and almonds.
2. Pour the dressing over the salad and lightly toss.
3. Divide into four equal portions and top each with sliced avocado and 1 tablespoon of crumbled feta (if using).

Make the Dressing

1. In a small bowl, whisk together the olive oil, honey, and balsamic vinegar.

Per Serving

calories: 339 | fat: 22g | protein: 25g | carbs: 13g | sugars: 6g | fiber: 6g | sodium: 132mg

Chicken, Cantaloupe, Kale, and Almond Salad

Prep time: 10 minutes | Cook time: 0 minutes | Serves 3

Salad:

4 cups chopped kale, packed
1½ cups diced cantaloupe
1½ cups shredded rotisserie chicken
½ cup sliced almonds
¼ cup crumbled feta

Dressing:

2 teaspoons honey
2 tablespoons extra-virgin olive oil
2 teaspoons apple
cider vinegar or freshly squeezed lemon juice

Make the Salad

1. Divide the kale into three portions. Layer ⅓ of the cantaloupe, chicken, almonds, and feta on each portion.
2. Drizzle some of the dressing over each portion of salad. Serve immediately.

Make the Dressing

1. In a small bowl, whisk together the honey, olive oil, and vinegar.

Per Serving

calories: 396 | fat:22 g | protein: 27g | carbs: 24g | sugars: 12g | fiber: 4g | sodium: 236mg

Chicken and Brussels Sprout Cobb Salad

Prep time: 10 minutes | Cook time: 30 minutes | Serves 4

Salad:

8 (2-ounce / 57-g) chicken tenders
Avocado oil cooking spray
2 slices turkey bacon
2 (9-ounce / 255-
g) packages shaved Brussels sprouts
2 hard-boiled eggs, chopped
½ cup unsweetened dried cranberries

Dressing:

3 tablespoons honey mustard
3 tablespoons extra-
virgin olive oil
½ tablespoon freshly squeezed lemon juice

Make the Salad

1. Preheat the oven to 425ºF (220ºC).
2. Lightly coat the chicken tenders with cooking spray, then place them on a baking sheet and bake for 15 to 18 minutes.
3. Meanwhile, heat a large skillet over medium-low heat. When hot, fry the bacon for 5 to 7 minutes until crispy. When the bacon is done, carefully remove it from the pan, and set it on a plate lined with a paper towel to drain and cool. Crumble when cool enough to handle.
4. Cut the chicken tenders into even pieces. Divide the Brussels sprouts into four equal portions. Top each portion with one-quarter of the chopped eggs, crumbled bacon, dried cranberries, and 2 sliced chicken tenders.
5. Drizzle an equal portion of dressing over each serving.

Make the Dressing

1. In a small bowl, whisk together the mustard, olive oil, and lemon juice.

Per Serving

calories: 468 | fat: 20g | protein: 35g | carbs: 37g | sugars: 14g | fiber: 10g | sodium: 242mg

Cabbage and Carrot Slaw

Prep time: 15 minutes | Cook time: 0 minutes | Serves 6

2 cups finely chopped green cabbage
2 cups finely chopped red cabbage
2 cups grated carrots
3 scallions, both white and green parts, sliced

2 tablespoons extra-virgin olive oil
2 tablespoons rice vinegar
1 teaspoon honey
1 garlic clove, minced
¼ teaspoon salt

1. In a large bowl, toss together the green and red cabbage, carrots, and scallions.
2. In a small bowl, whisk together the oil, vinegar, honey, garlic, and salt.
3. Pour the dressing over the veggies and mix to thoroughly combine.
4. Serve immediately, or cover and chill for several hours before serving.

Per Serving
calories: 80 | fat: 5g | protein: 1g | carbs: 10g | sugars: 6g | fiber: 3g | sodium: 126mg

Squash and Barley Salad

Prep time: 20 minutes | Cook time: 40 minutes | Serves 8

1 small butternut squash
3 teaspoons plus 2 tablespoons extra-virgin olive oil, divided
2 cups broccoli florets
1 cup pearl barley
1 cup toasted chopped walnuts

2 cups baby kale
½ red onion, sliced
2 tablespoons balsamic vinegar
2 garlic cloves, minced
½ teaspoon salt
¼ teaspoon freshly ground black pepper

1. Preheat the oven to 400ºF (205ºC). Line a baking sheet with parchment paper.
2. Peel and seed the squash, and cut it into dice. In a large bowl, toss the squash with 2 teaspoons of olive oil. Transfer to the prepared baking sheet and roast for 20 minutes.
3. While the squash is roasting, toss the broccoli in the same bowl with 1 teaspoon of olive oil. After 20 minutes, flip the squash and push it to one side of the baking sheet. Add the broccoli to the other side and continue to roast for 20 more minutes until tender.

4. While the veggies are roasting, in a medium pot, cover the barley with several inches of water. Bring to a boil, then reduce the heat, cover, and simmer for 30 minutes until tender. Drain and rinse.
5. Transfer the barley to a large bowl, and toss with the cooked squash and broccoli, walnuts, kale, and onion.
6. In a small bowl, mix the remaining 2 tablespoons of olive oil, balsamic vinegar, garlic, salt, and pepper. Toss the salad with the dressing and serve.

Per Serving
calories: 275 | fat: 15g | protein: 6g | carbs: 32g | sugars: 3g | fiber: 7g | sodium: 144mg

Savory Skillet Corn Bread

Prep time: 15 minutes | Cook time: 20 minutes | Serves 8

Nonstick cooking spray
1 cup whole-wheat all-purpose flour
1 cup yellow cornmeal
1¾ teaspoons baking powder
¾ teaspoon baking soda
½ teaspoon salt
1 large zucchini,

grated
1 cup reduced-fat Cheddar cheese, grated
¼ bunch chives, finely chopped
1 cup buttermilk
2 large eggs
3 tablespoons canola oil

1. Preheat the oven to 425ºF (220ºC). Lightly spray a cast iron skillet with cooking spray.
2. In a medium bowl, whisk the flour, cornmeal, baking powder, baking soda, and salt together.
3. In a large bowl, gently whisk the zucchini, cheese, chives, buttermilk, eggs, and oil together.
4. Add the dry ingredients to the wet ingredients, and stir until just combined, taking care not to overmix, and pour into the prepared skillet.
5. Transfer the skillet to the oven, and bake for 20 minutes, or until a knife inserted into the center comes out clean. Remove from the oven, and let sit for 10 minutes before serving.

Per Serving
calories: 235 | fat: 11g | protein: 9g | carbs: 27g | sugars: 2g | fiber: 2g | sodium: 340mg

Grilled Romaine with Buttermilk Dressing

Prep time: 5 minutes | Cook time: 5 minutes | Serves 4

Romaine:
2 heads romaine lettuce, halved lengthwise
2 tablespoons extra-virgin olive oil

Dressing:

½ cup low-fat buttermilk	¼ bunch fresh chives, thinly chopped
1 tablespoon extra-virgin olive oil	1 pinch red pepper flakes
1 garlic clove, pressed	

Make the Romaine
1. Heat a grill pan over medium heat.
2. Brush each lettuce half with the olive oil, and place flat-side down on the grill. Grill for 3 to 5 minutes, or until the lettuce slightly wilts and develops light grill marks.

Make the Dressing
1. In a small bowl, whisk the buttermilk, olive oil, garlic, chives, and red pepper flakes together.
2. Drizzle 2 tablespoons of dressing over each romaine half, and serve.

Per Serving
calories: 126 | fat: 11g | protein: 2g | carbs: 7g | sugars: 3g | fiber: 1g | sodium: 41mg

Parmesan Cauliflower Mash

Prep time: 7 minutes | Cook time: 5 minutes | Serves 4

1 head cauliflower, cored and cut into large florets	Greek yogurt
½ teaspoon kosher salt	¾ cup freshly grated Parmesan cheese
½ teaspoon garlic pepper	1 tablespoon unsalted butter or ghee (optional)
2 tablespoons plain	Chopped fresh chives

1. Pour 1 cup of water into the electric pressure cooker and insert a steamer basket or wire rack.
2. Place the cauliflower in the basket.
3. Close and lock the lid of the pressure cooker. Set the valve to sealing.
4. Cook on high pressure for 5 minutes.
5. When the cooking is complete, hit Cancel and quick release the pressure.

6. Once the pin drops, unlock and remove the lid.
7. Remove the cauliflower from the pot and pour out the water. Return the cauliflower to the pot and add the salt, garlic pepper, yogurt, and cheese. Use an immersion blender or potato masher to purée or mash the cauliflower in the pot.
8. Spoon into a serving bowl, and garnish with butter (if using) and chives.

Per Serving
calories: 141 | fat: 6g | protein: 12g | carbs: 12g | sugars: 5g | fiber: 4g | sodium: 592mg

Parmesan-Topped Acorn Squash

Prep time: 10 minutes | Cook time: 20 minutes | Serves 4

1 acorn squash (about 1 pound / 454 g)	⅛ teaspoon kosher salt
1 tablespoon extra-virgin olive oil	⅛ teaspoon freshly ground black pepper
1 teaspoon dried sage leaves, crumbled	2 tablespoons freshly grated Parmesan cheese
¼ teaspoon freshly grated nutmeg	

1. Cut the acorn squash in half lengthwise and remove the seeds. Cut each half in half for a total of 4 wedges. Snap off the stem if it's easy to do.
2. In a small bowl, combine the olive oil, sage, nutmeg, salt, and pepper. Brush the cut sides of the squash with the olive oil mixture.
3. Pour 1 cup of water into the electric pressure cooker and insert a wire rack or trivet.
4. Place the squash on the trivet in a single layer, skin-side down.
5. Close and lock the lid of the pressure cooker. Set the valve to sealing.
6. Cook on high pressure for 20 minutes.
7. When the cooking is complete, hit Cancel and quick release the pressure.
8. Once the pin drops, unlock and remove the lid.
9. Carefully remove the squash from the pot, sprinkle with the Parmesan, and serve.

Per Serving
calories: 85 | fat: 4g | protein: 2g | carbs: 12g | sugars: 0g | fiber: 2g | sodium: 282mg

Green Bean Casserole

Prep time: 10 minutes | Cook time: 30 minutes | Serves 8

1 pound (454 g) green beans, trimmed, cut into bite-size pieces
3 tablespoons extra-virgin olive oil, divided
8 ounces (227 g) brown mushrooms, diced
3 garlic cloves, minced
1½ tablespoons whole-wheat flour
1 cup low-sodium vegetable broth
1 cup unsweetened plain almond milk
¼ cup almond flour
2 tablespoons dried minced onion

1. Preheat the oven to 400ºF (205ºC).
2. Bring a large pot of water to a boil. Boil the green beans for 3 to 5 minutes until just barely tender but still bright green. Drain and set aside.
3. In a medium skillet, heat 2 tablespoons of oil over medium-high heat. Add the mushrooms and stir. Cook for 3 to 5 minutes until the mushrooms brown and release their liquid. Add the garlic and stir until just fragrant, about 30 seconds.
4. Add the whole-wheat flour and stir well to combine. Add the broth and simmer for 1 minute.
5. Reduce the heat to medium low and add the almond milk. Return to a simmer and cook for 5 to 7 minutes until the mixture thickens.
6. Remove from the heat. Stir in the green beans and transfer to a baking dish.
7. In a small bowl, mix the almond flour, dried minced onion, and remaining 1 tablespoon of olive oil, and stir until combined and crumbly. Crumble over the beans.
8. Bake for 15 to 20 minutes until the liquids are bubbling and the top is browned.

Per Serving
calories: 97 | fat: 7g | protein: 2g | carbs: 7g | sugars: 2g | fiber: 2g | sodium: 57mg

Strawberry Farro Salad

Prep time: 17 minutes | Cook time: 10 minutes | Serves 8

Farro:
1 cup farro, rinsed and drained
¼ teaspoon kosher salt
Dressing:
1 tablespoon freshly squeezed lime juice (from ½ medium lime)
½ tablespoon fruit-flavored balsamic vinegar
½ teaspoon Dijon mustard
½ tablespoon honey or pure maple syrup
½ teaspoon poppy seeds
¼ cup extra-virgin olive oil
Salad:
1¼ cups sliced strawberries
¼ cup slivered almonds, toasted
Freshly ground black pepper, to taste
Fresh basil leaves, cut into a chiffonade, for garnish

Make the Farro
1. In the electric pressure cooker, combine the farro, salt, and 2 cups of water.
2. Close and lock the lid. Set the valve to sealing.
3. Cook on high pressure for 10 minutes.
4. When the cooking is complete, allow the pressure to release naturally for 10 minutes, then quick release the remaining pressure. Hit Cancel.
5. Once the pin drops, unlock and remove the lid.
6. Fluff the farro with a fork and let cool.

Make the Dressing
1. While the farro is cooking, in a small jar with a screw-top lid, combine the lime juice, balsamic vinegar, mustard, honey, poppy seeds, and olive oil. Shake until well combined.
2. Make the Salad
3. In a large bowl, toss the farro with the dressing. Stir in the strawberries and almonds.
4. Season with pepper, garnish with basil, and serve.

Per Serving (½ cup)
calories: 176 | fat: 9g | protein: 3g | carbs: 22g | sugars: 3g | fiber: 2g | sodium: 68mg

Quinoa, Salmon, and Avocado Salad

Prep time: 15 minutes | Cook time: 20 minutes | Serves 4

½ cup quinoa
1 cup water
4 (4-ounce / 113-g) salmon fillets
1 pound (454 g) asparagus, trimmed
1 teaspoon extra-virgin olive oil, plus 2 tablespoons
½ teaspoon salt, divided
½ teaspoon freshly ground black pepper, divided
¼ teaspoon red pepper flakes
1 avocado, chopped
¼ cup chopped scallions, both white and green parts
¼ cup chopped fresh cilantro
1 tablespoon minced fresh oregano
Juice of 1 lime

1. In a small pot, combine the quinoa and water, and bring to a boil over medium-high heat. Cover, reduce the heat, and simmer for 15 minutes.
2. Preheat the oven to 425ºF (220ºC). Line a large baking sheet with parchment paper.
3. Arrange the salmon on one side of the prepared baking sheet. Toss the asparagus with 1 teaspoon of olive oil, and arrange on the other side of the baking sheet. Season the salmon and asparagus with ¼ teaspoon of salt, ¼ teaspoon of pepper, and the red pepper flakes. Roast for 12 minutes until browned and cooked through.
4. While the fish and asparagus are cooking, in a large mixing bowl, gently toss the cooked quinoa, avocado, scallions, cilantro, and oregano. Add the remaining 2 tablespoons of olive oil and the lime juice, and season with the remaining ¼ teaspoon of salt and ¼ teaspoon of pepper.
5. Break the salmon into pieces, removing the skin and any bones, and chop the asparagus into bite-sized pieces. Fold into the quinoa and serve warm or at room temperature.

Per Serving
calories: 397 | fat: 22g | protein: 29g | carbs: 23g | sugars: 3g | fiber: 8g | sodium: 292mg

Lemony Black Rice Salad with Edamame

Prep time: 15 minutes | Cook time: 22 minutes | Serves 8

Rice:
1 cup black rice (forbidden rice), rinsed and still wet
Dressing:
3 tablespoons extra-virgin olive oil
2 tablespoons freshly squeezed lemon juice
2 tablespoons white wine vinegar or rice vinegar
1 tablespoon honey or pure maple syrup
1 tablespoon sesame oil
Salad:
1 (8-ounce / 227-g) bag frozen shelled edamame, thawed (about 1½ cups)
2 scallions, both white and green parts, thinly sliced
¼ cup chopped walnuts
Kosher salt and freshly ground black pepper, to taste

Make the Rice
1. In the electric pressure cooker, combine the rice and 1 cup of water.
2. Close and lock the lid of the pressure cooker. Set the valve to sealing.
3. Cook on high pressure for 22 minutes.
4. When the cooking is complete, hit Cancel and allow the pressure to release naturally for 10 minutes, then quick release any remaining pressure.
5. Once the pin drops, unlock and remove the lid.
6. Fluff the rice with a fork and let it cool.

Make the Dressing
1. While the rice is cooking, make the dressing. In a small jar with a screw-top lid, combine the olive oil, lemon juice, vinegar, honey or maple syrup, and sesame oil. Shake until well combined.
2. Make the Salad
3. Shake up the dressing. In a large bowl, toss the rice and dressing. Stir in the edamame, scallions, and walnuts.
4. Season with salt and pepper.

Per Serving (½ cup)
calories: 170 | fat: 11g | protein: 5g | carbs: 15g | sugars: 3g | fiber: 2g | sodium: 10mg

Lemony Brussels Sprouts with Poppy Seeds

Prep time: 10 minutes | Cook time: 2 minutes | Serves 4

1 pound (454 g) Brussels sprouts	½ teaspoon kosher salt
2 tablespoons avocado oil, divided	Freshly ground black pepper, to taste
1 cup vegetable broth or chicken bone broth	½ medium lemon
1 tablespoon minced garlic	½ tablespoon poppy seeds

1. Trim the Brussels sprouts by cutting off the stem ends and removing any loose outer leaves. Cut each in half lengthwise (through the stem).
2. Set the electric pressure cooker to the Sauté/More setting. When the pot is hot, pour in 1 tablespoon of the avocado oil.
3. Add half of the Brussels sprouts to the pot, cut-side down, and let them brown for 3 to 5 minutes without disturbing. Transfer to a bowl and add the remaining tablespoon of avocado oil and the remaining Brussels sprouts to the pot. Hit Cancel and return all of the Brussels sprouts to the pot.
4. Add the broth, garlic, salt, and a few grinds of pepper. Stir to distribute the seasonings.
5. Close and lock the lid of the pressure cooker. Set the valve to sealing.
6. Cook on high pressure for 2 minutes.
7. While the Brussels sprouts are cooking, zest the lemon, then cut it into quarters.
8. When the cooking is complete, hit Cancel and quick release the pressure.
9. Once the pin drops, unlock and remove the lid.
10. Using a slotted spoon, transfer the Brussels sprouts to a serving bowl. Toss with the lemon zest, a squeeze of lemon juice, and the poppy seeds. Serve immediately.

Per Serving
calories: 125 | fat: 8g | protein: 4g | carbs: 13g | sugars: 3g | fiber: 5g | sodium: 504mg

Rice Salad with Cranberries and Almonds

Prep time: 10 minutes | Cook time: 25 minutes | Serves 18

Rice:

2 cups wild rice blend, rinsed	2½ cups vegetable broth or chicken bone broth
1 teaspoon kosher salt	

Dressing:

¼ cup extra-virgin olive oil	orange zest
¼ cup white wine vinegar	Juice of 1 medium orange (about ¼ cup)
1½ teaspoons grated	1 teaspoon honey or pure maple syrup

Salad:
¾ cup unsweetened dried cranberries
½ cup sliced almonds, toasted
Freshly ground black pepper, to taste

Make the Rice
1. In the electric pressure cooker, combine the rice, salt, and broth.
2. Close and lock the lid. Set the valve to sealing.
3. Cook on high pressure for 25 minutes.
4. When the cooking is complete, hit Cancel and allow the pressure to release naturally for 15 minutes, then quick release any remaining pressure.
5. Once the pin drops, unlock and remove the lid.
6. Let the rice cool briefly, then fluff it with a fork.

Make the Dressing
1. While the rice cooks, make the dressing: In a small jar with a screw-top lid, combine the olive oil, vinegar, zest, juice, and honey. (If you don't have a jar, whisk the ingredients together in a small bowl.) Shake to combine.
2. Make the Salad
3. In a large bowl, combine the rice, cranberries, and almonds.
4. Add the dressing and season with pepper.
5. Serve warm or refrigerate.

Per Serving (¹⁄₃ cup)
calories: 126 | fat: 5g | protein: 3g | carbs: 18g | sugars: 2g | fiber: 2g | sodium: 120mg

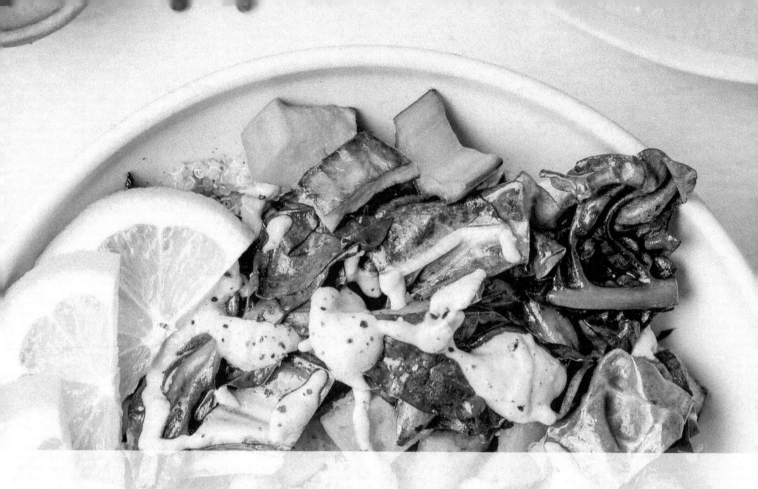

Chapter 5 Meatless Mains

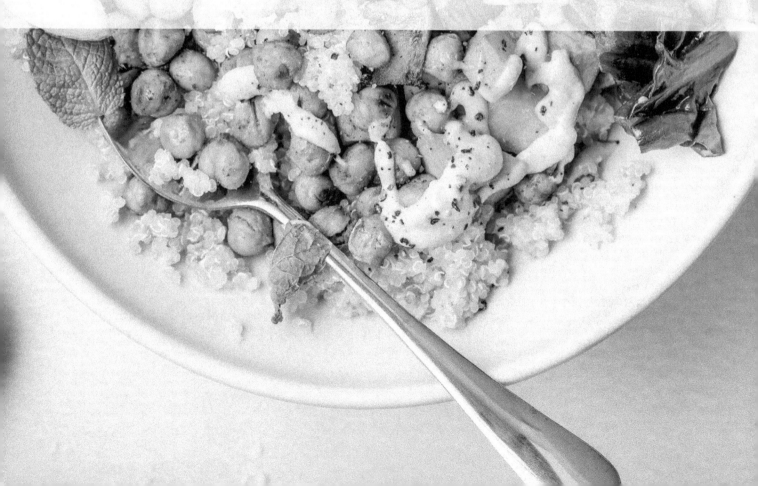

Mushroom and Cauliflower Rice Risotto

Prep time: 5 minutes | Cook time: 10 minutes | Serves 4

1 teaspoon extra-virgin olive oil
½ cup chopped portobello mushrooms
4 cups cauliflower rice
¼ cup low-sodium vegetable broth
½ cup half-and-half
1 cup shredded Parmesan cheese

1. Heat the oil in a medium skillet over medium-low heat. When hot, put the mushrooms in the skillet and cook for 3 minutes, stirring once.
2. Add the cauliflower rice, broth, and half-and-half. Stir and cover. Increase to high heat and boil for 5 minutes.
3. Add the cheese. Stir to incorporate. Cook for 3 more minutes.

Per Serving

calories: 168 | fat: 11g | protein: 12g | carbs: 8g | sugars: 4g | fiber: 3g | sodium: 327mg

Stuffed Portobello Mushrooms

Prep time: 5 minutes | Cook time: 20 minutes | Serves 4

8 large portobello mushrooms
3 teaspoons extra-virgin olive oil, divided
4 cups fresh spinach
1 medium red bell pepper, diced
¼ cup crumbled feta

1. Preheat the oven to 450ºF (235ºC).
2. Remove the stems from the mushrooms, and gently scoop out the gills and discard. Coat the mushrooms with 2 teaspoons of olive oil.
3. On a baking sheet, place the mushrooms cap-side down, and roast for 20 minutes.
4. Meanwhile, heat the remaining 1 teaspoon of olive oil in a medium skillet over medium heat. When hot, sauté the spinach and red bell pepper for 8 to 10 minutes, stirring occasionally.
5. Remove the mushrooms from the oven. Drain, if necessary. Spoon the spinach and pepper mix into the mushrooms, and top with feta.

Per Serving

calories: 116 | fat: 6g | protein: 7g | carbs: 12g | sugars: 6g | fiber: 4g | sodium: 126mg

No-Tuna Lettuce Wraps

Prep time: 10 minutes | Cook time: 0 minutes | Serves 4

1 (15-ounce / 425-g) can low-sodium chickpeas, drained and rinsed
1 celery stalk, thinly sliced
3 tablespoons honey mustard
2 tablespoons finely chopped red onion
2 tablespoons unsalted tahini
1 tablespoon capers, undrained
12 butter lettuce leaves

1. In a large bowl, mash the chickpeas.
2. Add the celery, honey mustard, onion, tahini, and capers, and mix well.
3. For each serving, place three lettuce leaves on a plate so they overlap, top with one-fourth of the chickpea filling, and roll up into a wrap. Repeat with the remaining lettuce leaves and filling.

Per Serving

calories: 183 | fat: 7g | protein: 10g | carbs: 20g | sugars: 9g | fiber: 3g | sodium: 172mg

Italian Zucchini Boats

Prep time: 5 minutes | Cook time: 15 minutes | Serves 4

1 cup canned low-sodium chickpeas, drained and rinsed
1 cup no-sugar-added spaghetti sauce
2 zucchini
¼ cup shredded Parmesan cheese

1. Preheat the oven to 425ºF (220ºC).
2. In a medium bowl, mix the chickpeas and spaghetti sauce together.
3. Cut the zucchini in half lengthwise, and scrape a spoon gently down the length of each half to remove the seeds.
4. Fill each zucchini half with the chickpea sauce, and top with one-quarter of the Parmesan cheese.
5. Place the zucchini halves on a baking sheet and roast in the oven for 15 minutes.

Per Serving

calories: 139 | fat: 4g | protein: 8g | carbs: 20g | sugars: 6g | fiber: 5g | sodium: 344mg

Pizza Stuffed Pita

Prep time: 10 minutes | Cook time: 0 minutes | Serves 2

½ cup tomato sauce
½ teaspoon oregano
½ teaspoon garlic powder
½ cup chopped black olives
2 canned artichoke hearts, drained and

chopped
2 ounces (57 g) pepperoni, chopped
½ cup shredded Mozzarella cheese
1 whole-wheat pita, halved

1. In a medium bowl, stir together the tomato sauce, oregano, and garlic powder.
2. Add the olives, artichoke hearts, pepperoni, and cheese. Stir to mix.
3. Spoon the mixture into the pita halves.

Per Serving

calories: 376 | fat: 23g | protein: 17g | carbs: 27g | sugars: 8g | fiber: 6g | sodium: 1076mg

Tofu Veggie Stir-Fry

Prep time: 10 minutes | Cook time: 20 minutes | Serves 4

3 tablespoons extra-virgin olive oil
4 scallions, sliced
12 ounces (340 g) firm tofu, cut into ½-inch pieces
4 cups broccoli, broken into florets
4 garlic cloves, minced
1 teaspoon peeled

and grated fresh ginger
¼ cup vegetable broth
2 tablespoons soy sauce (use gluten-free soy sauce if necessary)
1 cup cooked brown rice

1. In a large skillet over medium-high heat, heat the olive oil until it shimmers. Add the scallions, tofu, and broccoli and cook, stirring, until the vegetables begin to soften, about 6 minutes. Add the garlic and ginger and cook, stirring constantly, for 30 seconds.
2. Add the broth, soy sauce, and rice. Cook, stirring, 1 to 2 minutes more to heat the rice through.

Per Serving

calories: 236 | fat: 13g | protein: 11g | carbs: 21g | sugars: 0g | fiber: 4g | sodium: 361mg

Bulgur and Eggplant Pilaf

Prep time: 10 minutes | Cook time: 1 hour | Serves 4

½ sweet onion, chopped
2 teaspoons minced garlic
1 cup chopped eggplant
1½ cups bulgur
4 cups low-sodium

chicken broth
1 cup diced tomato
Sea salt and freshly ground black pepper, to taste
2 tablespoons chopped fresh basil

1. Place a large saucepan over medium-high heat. Add the oil and sauté the onion and garlic until softened and translucent, about 3 minutes.
2. Stir in the eggplant and sauté 4 minutes to soften.
3. Stir in the bulgur, broth, and tomatoes. Bring the mixture to a boil.
4. Reduce the heat to low, cover, and simmer until the water has been absorbed, about 50 minutes.
5. Season the pilaf with salt and pepper.
6. Garnish with the basil, and serve.

Per Serving

calories: 297 | fat: 4g | protein: 14g | carbs: 54g | sugars: 7g | fiber: 12g | sodium: 357mg

Egg Salad Wraps

Prep time: 10 minutes | Cook time: 0 minutes | Serves 2

3 tablespoons mayonnaise
1 teaspoon Dijon mustard
1 tablespoon chopped fresh dill
½ teaspoon sea salt
¼ teaspoon paprika

4 hard-boiled large eggs, chopped
1 cup shelled fresh peas
2 tablespoons finely chopped red onion
2 large kale leaves

1. In a medium bowl, whisk together the mayonnaise, mustard, dill, salt, and paprika.
2. Stir in the eggs, peas, and onion.
3. Serve wrapped in kale leaves.

Per Serving

calories: 296 | fat: 18g | protein: 17g | carbs: 18g | sugars: 2g | fiber: 4g | sodium: 620mg

Zoodles with Beet and Walnut Pesto

Prep time: 15 minutes | Cook time: 40 minutes | Serves 2

1 medium red beet, peeled, chopped
½ cup walnut pieces
3 garlic cloves
½ cup crumbled goat cheese
2 tablespoons extra-

virgin olive oil, plus 2 teaspoons
2 tablespoons freshly squeezed lemon juice
¼ teaspoon salt
4 small zucchini

1. Preheat the oven to 375ºF (190ºC).
2. Wrap the chopped beet in a piece of aluminum foil and seal well. Roast for 30 to 40 minutes until fork-tender.
3. Meanwhile, heat a dry skillet over medium-high heat. Toast the walnuts for 5 to 7 minutes until lightly browned and fragrant.
4. Transfer the cooked beets to the bowl of a food processor. Add the toasted walnuts, garlic, goat cheese, 2 tablespoons of olive oil, lemon juice, and salt. Process until smooth.
5. Using a spiralizer or sharp knife, cut the zucchini into thin "noodles."
6. In a large skillet, heat the remaining 2 teaspoons of oil over medium heat. Add the zucchini and toss in the oil. Cook, stirring gently, for 2 to 3 minutes, until the zucchini softens. Toss with the beet pesto and serve warm.

Per Serving
calories: 422 | fat: 39g | protein: 8g | carbs: 17g | sugars: 10g | fiber: 6g | sodium: 339mg

Open-Faced Egg Salad Sandwiches

Prep time: 10 minutes | Cook time: 0 minutes | Serves 4

8 large hard-boiled eggs
3 tablespoons plain low-fat Greek yogurt
1 tablespoon mustard
½ teaspoon freshly ground black pepper

1 teaspoon chopped fresh chives
4 slices 100% whole-wheat bread
2 cups fresh spinach, loosely packed

1. Peel the eggs and cut them in half.
2. In a large bowl, mash the eggs with a fork, leaving chunks.
3. Add the yogurt, mustard, pepper, and chives, and mix.
4. For each portion, layer 1 slice of bread with one-quarter of the egg salad and spinach.

Per Serving
calories: 277 | fat: 12g | protein: 20g | carbs: 23g | sugars: 3g | fiber: 3g | sodium: 364mg

Stuffed Squash with Cheese and Artichokes

Prep time: 10 minutes | Cook time: 45 minutes | Serves 4

1 small spaghetti squash, halved and seeded
½ cup low-fat cottage cheese
¼ cup shredded Mozzarella cheese, divided
2 garlic cloves,

minced
1 cup artichoke hearts, chopped
1 cup thinly sliced kale
⅛ teaspoon salt
Pinch freshly ground black pepper

1. Preheat the oven to 400ºF (205ºC). Line a baking sheet with parchment paper.
2. Place the cut squash halves on the prepared baking sheet cut-side down, and roast for 30 to 40 minutes, depending on the size and thickness of the squash, until they are fork-tender. Set aside to cool slightly.
3. In a large bowl, mix the cottage cheese, 2 tablespoons of Mozzarella cheese, garlic, artichoke hearts, kale, salt, and pepper.
4. Preheat the broiler to high.
5. Using a fork, break apart the flesh of the spaghetti squash into strands, being careful to leave the skin intact. Add the strands to the cheese and vegetable mixture. Toss gently to combine.
6. Divide the mixture between the two hollowed-out squash halves and top with the remaining 2 tablespoons of cheese.
7. Broil for 5 to 7 minutes until browned and heated through.
8. Cut each piece of stuffed squash in half to serve.

Per Serving
calories: 142 | fat: 4g | protein: 9g | carbs: 19g | sugars: 10g | fiber: 4g | sodium: 312mg

Mushroom Pesto Flatbread Pizza

Prep time: 5 minutes | Cook time: 15 minutes | Serves 2

1 teaspoon extra-virgin olive oil
½ cup sliced mushrooms
½ red onion, sliced
Salt and freshly ground black pepper,
to taste
¼ cup store-bought pesto sauce
2 whole-wheat flatbreads
¼ cup shredded Mozzarella cheese

1. Preheat the oven to 350ºF (180ºC).
2. In a small skillet, heat the oil over medium heat. Add the mushrooms and onion, and season with salt and pepper. Sauté for 3 to 5 minutes until the onion and mushrooms begin to soften.
3. Spread 2 tablespoons of pesto on each flatbread.
4. Divide the mushroom-onion mixture between the two flatbreads. Top each with 2 tablespoons of cheese.
5. Place the flatbreads on a baking sheet, and bake for 10 to 12 minutes until the cheese is melted and bubbly. Serve warm.

Per Serving

calories: 347 | fat: 23g | protein: 14g | carbs: 28g | sugars: 4g | fiber: 7g | sodium: 791mg

Vegetarian Black Bean Enchilada Skillet

Prep time: 15 minutes | Cook time: 15 minutes | Serves 6

1 tablespoon extra-virgin olive oil
½ onion, chopped
½ red bell pepper, seeded and chopped
½ green bell pepper, seeded and chopped
2 small zucchini, chopped
3 garlic cloves, minced
1 (15-ounce / 425-g) can low-sodium black beans, drained and rinsed
1 (10-ounce / 283-g) can low-sodium
enchilada sauce
1 teaspoon ground cumin
¼ teaspoon salt
¼ teaspoon freshly ground black pepper
½ cup shredded Cheddar cheese, divided
2 (6-inch) corn tortillas, cut into strips
Chopped fresh cilantro, for garnish
Plain yogurt, for serving

1. Heat the broiler to high.
2. In a large oven-safe skillet, heat the oil over medium-high heat.
3. Add the onion, red bell pepper, green bell pepper, zucchini, and garlic to the skillet, and cook for 3 to 5 minutes until the onion softens.
4. Add the black beans, enchilada sauce, cumin, salt, pepper, ¼ cup of cheese, and tortilla strips, and mix together. Top with the remaining ¼ cup of cheese.
5. Put the skillet under the broiler and broil for 5 to 8 minutes until the cheese is melted and bubbly. Garnish with cilantro and serve with yogurt on the side.

Per Serving

calories: 171 | fat: 7g | protein: 8g | carbs: 21g | sugars: 3g | fiber: 7g | sodium: 565mg

Brussels Sprouts Wild Rice Bowl

Prep time: 15 minutes | Cook time: 15 minutes | Serves 4

2 cups sliced Brussels sprouts
2 teaspoons extra-virgin olive oil, plus 2 tablespoons
Juice of 1 lemon
1 teaspoon Dijon mustard
1 garlic clove, minced
½ teaspoon salt
¼ teaspoon freshly ground black pepper
1 cup cooked wild rice
1 cup sliced radishes
1 avocado, sliced

1. Preheat the oven to 400ºF (205ºC). Line a baking sheet with parchment paper.
2. In a medium bowl, toss the Brussels sprouts with 2 teaspoons of olive oil and spread on the prepared baking sheet. Roast for 12 minutes, stirring once, until lightly browned.
3. In a small bowl, mix the remaining 2 tablespoons of olive oil, lemon juice, mustard, garlic, salt, and pepper.
4. In a large bowl, toss the cooked wild rice, radishes, and roasted Brussels sprouts. Drizzle the dressing over the salad and toss.
5. Divide among 4 bowls and top with avocado slices.

Per Serving

calories: 178 | fat: 11g | protein: 2g | carbs: 18g | sugars: 2g | fiber: 5g | sodium: 299mg

Texas Caviar

Prep time: 10 minutes | Cook time: 0 minutes | Serves 6

1 cup cooked black-eyed peas
1 cup cooked lima beans
1 ear fresh corn, kernels removed
2 celery stalks, chopped
1 red bell pepper, chopped
½ red onion, chopped
3 tablespoons apple cider vinegar
2 tablespoons extra-virgin olive oil
1 teaspoon paprika

1. In a large bowl, combine the black-eyed peas, lima beans, corn, celery, bell pepper, and onion.
2. In a small bowl, to make the dressing, whisk the vinegar, oil, and paprika together.
3. Pour the dressing over the bean mixture, and gently mix. Set aside for 15 to 30 minutes, allowing the flavors to come together.

Per Serving

calories: 170 | fat: 5g | protein: 10g | carbs: 29g | sugars: 4g | fiber: 10g | sodium: 20mg

Baked Vegetable Macaroni Pie

Prep time: 15 minutes | Cook time: 35 minutes | Serves 6

1 (16-ounce / 454-g) package whole-wheat macaroni
1 small yellow onion, chopped
2 garlic cloves, minced
2 celery stalks, thinly sliced
¼ teaspoon freshly ground black pepper
2 tablespoons
chickpea flour
1 cup fat-free milk
2 cups grated reduced-fat sharp Cheddar cheese
2 large zucchini, finely grated and squeezed dry
2 roasted red peppers, chopped into ¼-inch pieces

1. Preheat the oven to 350ºF (180ºC).
2. Bring a large pot of water to a boil.
3. Add the macaroni and cook for 2 to 5 minutes, or until al dente.
4. Drain the macaroni, reserving 1 cup of the pasta water for the cheese sauce. Rinse under cold running water, and transfer to a large bowl.
5. In a large cast iron skillet, warm the pasta water over medium heat.
6. Add the onion, garlic, celery, and pepper. Cook for 3 to 5 minutes, or until the onion is translucent.
7. Add the chickpea flour slowly, mixing often.
8. Stir in the milk and cheese until a thick liquid is formed. It should be about the consistency of a smoothie.
9. Add the pasta to the cheese mixture along with the zucchini and red peppers. Mix thoroughly so the ingredients are evenly dispersed.
10. Cover the skillet tightly with aluminum foil, transfer to the oven, and bake for 15 to 20 minutes, or until the cheese is well melted.
11. Uncover and bake for 5 minutes, or until golden brown.

Per Serving

calories: 378 | fat: 4g | protein: 24g | carbs: 67g | sugars: 6g | fiber: 8g| sodium: 332mg

Wild Rice with Blueberries and Pumpkin Seeds

Prep time: 15 minutes | Cook time: 45 minutes | Serves 4

1 tablespoon extra-virgin olive oil
½ sweet onion, chopped
2½ cups sodium-free chicken broth
1 cup wild rice, rinsed
and drained
Pinch sea salt
½ cup toasted pumpkin seeds
½ cup blueberries
1 teaspoon chopped fresh basil

1. Place a medium saucepan over medium-high heat and add the oil.
2. Sauté the onion until softened and translucent, about 3 minutes.
3. Stir in the broth and bring to a boil.
4. Stir in the rice and salt and reduce the heat to low. Cover and simmer until the rice is tender, about 40 minutes.
5. Drain off any excess broth, if necessary. Stir in the pumpkin seeds, blueberries, and basil.
6. Serve warm.

Per Serving

calories: 258 | fat: 9g | protein: 11g | carbs: 37g | sugars: 4g | fiber: 4g | sodium: 542mg

Herbed Beans and Brown Rice

Prep time: 15 minutes | Cook time: 15 minutes | Serves 8

2 teaspoons extra-virgin olive oil
½ sweet onion, chopped
1 teaspoon minced jalapeño pepper
1 teaspoon minced garlic
1 (15-ounce / 425-g) can sodium-free red kidney beans, rinsed
and drained
1 large tomato, chopped
1 teaspoon chopped fresh thyme
Sea salt and freshly ground black pepper, to taste
2 cups cooked brown rice

1. Place a large skillet over medium-high heat and add the olive oil.
2. Sauté the onion, jalapeño, and garlic until softened, about 3 minutes.
3. Stir in the beans, tomato, and thyme.
4. Cook until heated through, about 10 minutes. Season with salt and pepper.
5. Serve over the warm brown rice.

Per Serving

calories: 199 | fat: 2g | protein: 9g | carbs: 37g | sugars: 2g | fiber: 6g | sodium: 37mg

Mushroom Hazelnut Rice

Prep time: 20 minutes | Cook time: 35 minutes | Serves 8

1 tablespoon extra-virgin olive oil
1 cup chopped button mushrooms
½ sweet onion, chopped
1 celery stalk, chopped
2 teaspoons minced garlic
2 cups brown basmati
rice
4 cups low-sodium chicken broth
1 teaspoon chopped fresh thyme
Sea salt and freshly ground black pepper, to taste
½ cup chopped hazelnuts

1. Place a large saucepan over medium-high heat and add the oil.
2. Sauté the mushrooms, onion, celery, and garlic until lightly browned, about 10 minutes.
3. Add the rice and sauté for an additional minute.

4. Add the chicken broth and bring to a boil.
5. Reduce the heat to low and cover the pot. Simmer until the liquid is absorbed and the rice is tender, about 20 minutes.
6. Stir in the thyme and season with salt and pepper.
7. Top with the hazelnuts, and serve.

Per Serving

calories: 239 | fat: 6g | protein: 7g | carbs: 39g | sugars: 1g | fiber: 1g | sodium: 387mg

Quinoa Vegetable Skillet

Prep time: 15 minutes | Cook time: 15 minutes | Serves 6

2 cups vegetable broth
1 cup quinoa, well rinsed and drained
1 teaspoon extra-virgin olive oil
½ sweet onion, chopped
2 teaspoons minced garlic
½ large green zucchini, halved
lengthwise and cut into half disks
1 red bell pepper, seeded and cut into thin strips
1 cup fresh or frozen corn kernels
1 teaspoon chopped fresh basil
Sea salt and freshly ground black pepper, to taste

1. Place a medium saucepan over medium heat and add the vegetable broth. Bring the broth to a boil and add the quinoa. Cover and reduce the heat to low.
2. Cook until the quinoa has absorbed all the broth, about 15 minutes. Remove from the heat and let it cool slightly.
3. While the quinoa is cooking, place a large skillet over medium-high heat and add the oil.
4. Sauté the onion and garlic until softened and translucent, about 3 minutes.
5. Add the zucchini, bell pepper, and corn, and sauté until the vegetables are tender-crisp, about 5 minutes.
6. Remove the skillet from the heat. Add the cooked quinoa and the basil to the skillet, stirring to combine. Season with salt and pepper, and serve.

Per Serving

calories: 158 | fat: 3g | protein: 7g | carbs: 26g | sugars: 3g | fiber: 3g | sodium: 298mg

Ratatouille

Prep time: 10 minutes | Cook time: 30 minutes | Serves 4

4 tablespoons extra-virgin olive oil, divided
2 cups diced eggplant
1 cup diced zucchini
1 cup diced onion
1 cup chopped green bell pepper
1 (15-ounce / 425-g) can no-salt-added diced tomatoes
1 teaspoon ground thyme
½ teaspoon garlic powder
Salt and freshly ground black pepper, to taste

1. Heat a large saucepan over medium heat. When hot, heat 2 tablespoons of oil, then add the eggplant and the zucchini. Cook for 10 minutes, stirring occasionally. Watch to prevent burning because the eggplant will absorb the oil. Add the remaining 2 tablespoons of oil as necessary.
2. Add the onion and bell pepper, and cook for 5 minutes.
3. Add the diced tomatoes with their juices, thyme, and garlic powder, and cook for 15 minutes. Season with salt and pepper.

Per Serving

calories: 190 | fat: 14g | protein: 3g | carbs: 15g | sugars: 8g | fiber: 4g | sodium: 28mg

Ricotta Quinoa Bake

Prep time: 20 minutes | Cook time: 30 minutes | Serves 4

1 teaspoon extra-virgin olive oil
½ sweet onion, chopped
2 teaspoons minced garlic
2 cups cooked quinoa
2 eggs
½ cup low-fat ricotta cheese
Sea salt and freshly ground black pepper, to taste
2 cups cherry tomatoes
1 zucchini, cut into thin ribbons
⅛ cup pine nuts, toasted

1. Preheat the oven to 350ºF (180ºC).
2. Place a medium skillet over medium-high heat and add the olive oil.
3. Sauté the onion and garlic until softened and translucent, about 3 minutes.
4. Remove the skillet from the heat and stir in the quinoa, eggs, and ricotta.

5. Season the mixture with salt and pepper.
6. Stir in the cherry tomatoes and spoon the casserole into an 8-by-8-inch baking dish.
7. Scatter the zucchini ribbons and pine nuts on top, and bake the casserole until it is heated through, about 25 minutes.

Per Serving

calories: 302 | fat: 9g | protein: 17g | carbs: 38g | sugars: 5g | fiber: 4g | sodium: 234mg

Vegetarian Three-Bean Chili

Prep time: 20 minutes | Cook time: 1 hour | Serves 8

1 teaspoon extra-virgin olive oil
1 sweet onion, chopped
1 red bell pepper, seeded and diced
1 green bell pepper, seeded and diced
2 teaspoons minced garlic
1 (28-ounce / 794-g) can low-sodium diced tomatoes
1 (15-ounce / 425-g) can sodium-free black beans, rinsed and drained
1 (15-ounce / 425-g) can sodium-free red kidney beans, rinsed and drained
1 (15-ounce / 425-g) can sodium-free navy beans, rinsed and drained
2 tablespoons chili powder
2 teaspoons ground cumin
1 teaspoon ground coriander
¼ teaspoon red pepper flakes

1. Place a large saucepan over medium-high heat and add the oil.
2. Sauté the onion, red and green bell peppers, and garlic until the vegetables have softened, about 5 minutes.
3. Add the tomatoes, black beans, red kidney beans, navy beans, chili powder, cumin, coriander, and red pepper flakes to the pan.
4. Bring the chili to a boil, then reduce the heat to low.
5. Simmer the chili, stirring occasionally, for at least 1 hour.
6. Serve hot.

Per Serving

calories: 479 | fat: 28g | protein: 15g | carbs: 45g | sugars: 4g | fiber: 17g | sodium: 15mg

Salt-Free No-Soak Beans

Prep time: 2 minutes | Cook time: 25 to 40 minutes | Makes 6 cups

1 pound (454 g) dried beans, rinsed (unsoaked)
5 cups vegetable broth, chicken bone broth, or water
1 tablespoon extra-virgin olive oil

1. In the electric pressure cooker, combine the beans and broth. Drizzle the oil on top. (The oil will help control the foam produced by the cooking beans.)
2. Close and lock the lid of the pressure cooker. Set the valve to sealing.
3. For black beans, cook on high pressure for 25 minutes.
4. For pinto beans, navy beans, or great northern beans, cook on high pressure for 30 minutes.
5. For cannellini beans, cook on high pressure for 40 minutes.
6. When the cooking is complete, hit Cancel and allow the pressure to release naturally for 20 minutes, then quick release any remaining pressure.
7. Once the pin drops, unlock and remove the lid.
8. Let the beans cool, then pack them into containers and cover with the cooking liquid. Refrigerate for 3 to 5 days or freeze for up to 8 months.

Per Serving (½ cup)
calories: 141 | fat: 2g | protein: 8g | carbs: 24g | sugars: 1g | fiber: 6g | sodium: 5mg

Lentils with Carrots

Prep time: 15 minutes | Cook time: 12 minutes | Serves 6

2 tablespoons avocado oil
1 medium onion, chopped
3 celery stalks, chopped
1 teaspoon herbes de Provence
2 large carrots, chopped
2 cups vegetable broth or water
1 cup dried brown or green lentils, rinsed and drained
Kosher salt and freshly ground black pepper, to taste

1. Set the electric pressure cooker to the Sauté setting. When the pot is hot, pour in the avocado oil.

2. Sauté the onion and celery for 3 to 5 minutes, until the vegetables begin to soften. Stir in the herbes de Provence and carrots. Hit Cancel. Stir in the broth and lentils.
3. Close and lock the lid of the pressure cooker. Set the valve to sealing.
4. Cook on high pressure for 12 minutes.
5. When the cooking is complete, hit Cancel and allow the pressure to release naturally for 10 minutes, then quick release any remaining pressure.
6. Once the pin drops, unlock and remove the lid.
7. Season with salt and pepper, spoon into bowls, and serve.

Per Serving (⅔ cup)
calories: 178 | fat: 5g | protein: 9g | carbs: 24g | sugars: 3g | fiber: 11g | sodium: 45mg

Salt-Free Chickpeas (Garbanzo Beans)

Prep time: 5 minutes | Cook time: 35 minutes | Makes 6 cups

1 pound (454 g) dried chickpeas
2 bay leaves
Fresh herbs, like parsley, thyme, rosemary, etc., cut into 3-inch pieces and tied together with kitchen twine (optional)

1. Rinse the chickpeas and put them in the electric pressure cooker. Add 8 cups of water, the bay leaves, and the herbs (if using).
2. Close and lock the lid. Turn the pressure valve to sealing.
3. Cook on high pressure for 35 minutes.
4. When the cooking is complete, hit Cancel. Allow the pressure to release naturally for 20 minutes, then quick release any remaining pressure.
5. Unlock and remove the lid. Discard the bay leaves and herb bundle.
6. Transfer the chickpeas to storage containers, covered with the cooking liquid, and let cool. Refrigerate for 3 or 4 days or freeze for up to 6 months.

Per Serving (½ cup)
calories: 138 | fat: 2g | protein: 8g | carbs: 23g | sugars: 4g | fiber: 7g | sodium: 0mg

Chickpea and Tofu Bolognese

Prep time: 5 minutes | Cook time: 25 minutes | Serves 4

1 (3- to 4-pound / 1.4- to 1.8-kg) spaghetti squash
½ teaspoon ground cumin
1 cup no-sugar-added spaghetti sauce
1 (15-ounce / 425-g) can low-sodium chickpeas, drained and rinsed
6 ounces (170 g) extra-firm tofu

1. Preheat the oven to 400ºF (205ºC).
2. Cut the squash in half lengthwise. Scoop out the seeds and discard.
3. Season both halves of the squash with the cumin, and place them on a baking sheet cut-side down. Roast for 25 minutes.
4. Meanwhile, heat a medium saucepan over low heat, and pour in the spaghetti sauce and chickpeas.
5. Press the tofu between two layers of paper towels, and gently squeeze out any excess water.
6. Crumble the tofu into the sauce and cook for 15 minutes.
7. Remove the squash from the oven, and comb through the flesh of each half with a fork to make thin strands.
8. Divide the "spaghetti" into four portions, and top each portion with one-quarter of the sauce.

Per Serving
calories: 275 | fat: 7g | protein: 14g | carbs: 42g | sugars: 7g | fiber: 10g | sodium: 55mg

Spaghetti Puttanesca

Prep time: 20 minutes | Cook time: 35 minutes | Serves 6

1 tablespoon extra-virgin olive oil
1 sweet onion, chopped
2 celery stalks, chopped
3 teaspoons minced garlic
2 (28-ounce / 794-g) cans sodium-free diced tomatoes
2 tablespoons
chopped fresh basil
1 tablespoon chopped fresh oregano
½ teaspoon red pepper flakes
½ cup quartered, pitted Kalamata olives
¼ cup freshly squeezed lemon juice
8 ounces (227 g) whole-wheat spaghetti

1. Place a large saucepan over medium-high heat and add the oil.
2. Sauté the onion, celery, and garlic until they are translucent, about 3 minutes.
3. Add the tomatoes, basil, oregano, and red pepper flakes, and bring the sauce to a boil, stirring occasionally.
4. Reduce the heat to low and simmer 20 minutes, stirring occasionally.
5. Stir in the olives and lemon juice and remove the saucepan from the heat.
6. Cook the pasta according to the package instructions.
7. Spoon the sauce over the pasta and serve.

Per Serving
calories: 200 | fat: 5g | protein: 7g | carbs: 35g | sugars: 8g | fiber: 4g | sodium: 88mg

Tofu and Bean Chili

Prep time: 10 minutes | Cook time: 30 minutes | Serves 4

1 (15-ounce / 425-g) can low-sodium dark red kidney beans, drained and rinsed, divided
2 (15-ounce / 425-g) cans no-salt-added diced tomatoes
1½ cups low-sodium vegetable broth
½ teaspoon chili powder
½ teaspoon ground cumin
½ teaspoon garlic powder
½ teaspoon dried oregano
¼ teaspoon onion powder
¼ teaspoon salt
8 ounces (227 g) extra-firm tofu

1. In a small bowl, mash ⅓ of the beans with a fork.
2. Put the mashed beans, the remaining whole beans, and the diced tomatoes with their juices in a large stockpot.
3. Add the broth, chili powder, cumin, garlic powder, dried oregano, onion powder, and salt. Simmer over medium-high heat for 15 minutes.
4. Press the tofu between 3 or 4 layers of paper towels to squeeze out any excess moisture.
5. Crumble the tofu into the stockpot and stir. Simmer for another 10 to 15 minutes.

Per Serving
calories: 203 | fat: 3g | protein: 15g | carbs: 29g | sugars: 10g | fiber: 5g | sodium: 249mg

Chickpea Coconut Curry

Prep time: 5 minutes | Cook time: 15 minutes | Serves 4

3 cups fresh or frozen cauliflower florets
2 cups unsweetened almond milk
1 (15-ounce / 425-g) can coconut milk
1 (15-ounce / 425-g) can low-sodium chickpeas, drained and rinsed
1 tablespoon curry powder
¼ teaspoon ground ginger
¼ teaspoon garlic powder
⅛ teaspoon onion powder
¼ teaspoon salt

1. In a large stockpot, combine the cauliflower, almond milk, coconut milk, chickpeas, curry, ginger, garlic powder, and onion powder. Stir and cover.
2. Cook over medium-high heat for 10 minutes.
3. Reduce the heat to low, stir, and cook for 5 minutes more, uncovered. Season with up to ¼ teaspoon salt.

Per Serving
calories: 410 | fat: 30g | protein: 10g | carbs: 30g | sugars: 6g | fiber: 9g | sodium: 118mg

Cauliflower Steaks

Prep time: 5 minutes | Cook time: 20 minutes | Serves 4

Cauliflower:
1 head cauliflower
Avocado oil cooking spray
½ teaspoon garlic powder
4 cups arugula
Dressing:
1½ tablespoons honey mustard
1½ tablespoons extra-virgin olive oil
1 teaspoon freshly squeezed lemon juice

Make the Cauliflower
1. Preheat the oven to 425ºF (220ºC).
2. Remove the leaves from the cauliflower head, and cut it in half lengthwise.
3. Cut 1½-inch-thick steaks from each half.
4. Spray both sides of each steak with cooking spray, and season both sides with garlic powder.
5. Place the cauliflower steaks on a baking sheet, cover with foil, and roast for 10 minutes.

6. Remove the baking sheet from the oven and gently pull back the foil to avoid the steam. Flip the steaks, then roast uncovered for 10 minutes more.
7. Divide the cauliflower steaks into four equal portions. Top each portion with one-quarter of the arugula and dressing.

Make the Dressing
1. In a small bowl, whisk together the honey mustard, olive oil, and lemon juice.

Per Serving
calories: 115 | fat: 6g | protein: 5g | carbs: 14g | sugars: 6g | fiber: 4g | sodium: 97mg

Veggie Fajitas

Prep time: 10 minutes | Cook time: 15 minutes | Serves 4

Guacamole:
2 small avocados pitted and peeled
1 teaspoon freshly squeezed lime juice
¼ teaspoon salt
9 cherry tomatoes, halved
Fajitas:
1 red bell pepper
1 green bell pepper
1 small white onion
Avocado oil cooking spray
1 cup canned low-sodium black beans, drained and rinsed
½ teaspoon ground cumin
¼ teaspoon chili powder
¼ teaspoon garlic powder
4 (6-inch) yellow corn tortillas

Make the Guacamole
1. In a medium bowl, use a fork to mash the avocados with the lime juice and salt.
2. Gently stir in the cherry tomatoes.

Make the Fajitas
1. Cut the red bell pepper, green bell pepper, and onion into ½-inch slices.
2. Heat a large skillet over medium heat. When hot, coat the cooking surface with cooking spray. Put the peppers, onion, and beans into the skillet.
3. Add the cumin, chili powder, and garlic powder, and stir.
4. Cover and cook for 15 minutes, stirring halfway through.
5. Divide the fajita mixture equally between the tortillas, and top with guacamole and any preferred garnishes.

Per Serving
calories: 269 | fat: 15g | protein: 8g | carbs: 30g | sugars: 5g | fiber: 11g | sodium: 175mg

Almond Butter Apple Pita Pockets

Prep time: 10 minutes | Cook time: 0 minutes | Serves 2

½ apple, cored and chopped
¼ cup almond butter
½ teaspoon cinnamon
1 whole-wheat pita, halved

1. In a medium bowl, stir together the apple, almond butter, and cinnamon.
2. Spread with a spoon into the pita pocket halves.

Per Serving
calories: 313 | fat: 20g | protein: 8g | carbs: 31g | sugars: 6g | fiber: 7g | sodium: 174mg

Spinach Mini Crustless Quiches

Prep time: 10 minutes | Cook time: 15 minutes | Serves 6

Nonstick cooking spray
2 tablespoons extra-virgin olive oil
1 onion, finely chopped
2 cups baby spinach
2 garlic cloves, minced
8 large eggs, beaten
¼ cup whole milk
½ teaspoon sea salt
¼ teaspoon freshly ground black pepper
1 cup shredded Swiss cheese

1. Preheat the oven to 375ºF (190ºC). Spray a 6-cup muffin tin with nonstick cooking spray.
2. In a large skillet over medium-high heat, heat the olive oil until it shimmers. Add the onion and cook until soft, about 4 minutes. Add the spinach and cook, stirring, until the spinach softens, about 1 minute. Add the garlic. Cook, stirring constantly, for 30 seconds. Remove from heat and let cool.
3. In a medium bowl, beat together the eggs, milk, salt, and pepper.
4. Fold the cooled vegetables and the cheese into the egg mixture. Spoon the mixture into the prepared muffin tins. Bake until the eggs are set, about 15 minutes. Allow to rest for 5 minutes before serving.

Per Serving
calories: 218 | fat: 17g | protein: 14g | carbs: 4g | sugars: 3g | fiber: 0g | sodium: 237mg

Baked Tofu and Mixed Vegetable Bowl

Prep time: 10 minutes | Cook time: 20 minutes | Serves 4

Nonstick cooking spray
1 (14-ounce / 397-g) container firm tofu, cut into 1½-inch cubes
2 tablespoons low-sodium gluten-free soy sauce or tamari
1 tablespoon toasted sesame oil
1 teaspoon grated fresh ginger
1 teaspoon honey
2 garlic cloves, minced
2 teaspoons cornstarch
¼ cup water, plus 2 tablespoons
2 teaspoons extra-virgin olive oil
2 cups thinly sliced bok choy
1 cup sliced shiitake mushrooms
1 cup thinly sliced carrots
1 (14-ounce / 397-g) can baby corn, drained and rinsed
4 scallions, both white and green parts, chopped

1. Preheat the oven to 400ºF (205ºC). Line a baking sheet with parchment paper. Spray the parchment paper with nonstick cooking spray.
2. Place the tofu cubes on the prepared baking sheet and bake for 20 minutes, flipping once, until they are browned.
3. In a small bowl, combine the soy sauce, sesame oil, ginger, honey, and garlic. Stir well to combine.
4. In another small bowl, mix the cornstarch with ¼ cup of water and stir to combine. Add the soy sauce mixture, stir together, and set aside.
5. In a large skillet, heat the oil over medium heat. Add the boy choy, mushrooms, and carrots, and cook for 3 minutes, stirring regularly. Add the remaining 2 tablespoons of water, cover, and steam the vegetables for 3 more minutes until just fork-tender. Add the baby corn.
6. Pour the sauce and cooked tofu into the skillet, and bring to a boil. Reduce the heat and simmer for 1 to 2 minutes until the sauce thickens.
7. Divide the tofu and vegetables among 4 bowls. Top with scallions and serve.

Per Serving
calories: 212 | fat: 11g | protein: 12g | carbs: 22g | sugars: 7g | fiber: 4g | sodium: 526mg

Butternut Noodles with Mushroom Sauce

Prep time: 10 minutes | Cook time: 20 minutes | Serves 4

¼ cup extra-virgin olive oil
1 pound (454 g) cremini mushrooms, sliced
½ red onion, finely chopped
1 teaspoon dried thyme
½ teaspoon sea salt
3 garlic cloves, minced
½ cup dry white wine
Pinch red pepper flakes
4 cups butternut noodles
4 ounces (113 g) grated Parmesan cheese (optional, for serving)

1. In a large skillet over medium-high heat, heat the olive oil until it shimmers. Add the mushrooms, onion, thyme, and salt. Cook, stirring occasionally, until the mushrooms start to brown, about 6 minutes. Add the garlic and cook, stirring constantly, for 30 seconds. Add the white wine and red pepper flakes. Stir to combine.
2. Add the noodles. Cook, stirring occasionally, until the noodles are tender, about 5 minutes.
3. If desired, serve topped with grated Parmesan.

Per Serving
calories: 244 | fat: 14g | protein: 4g | carbs: 22g | sugars: 2g | fiber: 4g | sodium: 159mg

Tabbouleh Pita

Prep time: 20 minutes | Cook time: 0 minutes | Serves 4

4 whole-wheat pitas
1 cup cooked bulgur wheat
1 English cucumber, finely chopped
2 cups halved cherry tomatoes
1 yellow bell pepper, seeded and finely chopped
2 scallions, white and green parts, finely chopped
½ cup finely chopped fresh parsley
2 tablespoons extra-virgin olive oil
Juice of 1 lemon
Sea salt and freshly ground black pepper, to taste

1. Cut the pitas in half and split them open. Set them aside.
2. In a large bowl, stir together the bulgur, cucumber, tomatoes, bell pepper, scallions, parsley, olive oil, and lemon juice.
3. Season the bulgur mixture with salt and pepper.
4. Spoon the bulgur mixture evenly into the pita halves and serve.

Per Serving
calories: 242 | fat: 8g | protein: 7g | carbs: 39g | sugars: 4g | fiber: 6g | sodium: 164mg

Sweet Potato Kale Chickpea Bowl

Prep time: 10 minutes | Cook time: 15 minutes | Serves 2

Sauce:
2 tablespoons plain nonfat Greek yogurt
1 tablespoon tahini
2 tablespoons hemp seeds
1 garlic clove, minced
Pinch salt
Freshly ground black pepper, to taste

Bowl:
1 small sweet potato, peeled and finely diced
1 teaspoon extra-virgin olive oil
1 cup from 1
(15-ounce / 425-g) can low-sodium chickpeas, drained and rinsed
2 cups baby kale

Make the Sauce
1. In a small bowl, whisk together the yogurt and tahini.
2. Stir in the hemp seeds, garlic, and salt. Season with pepper. Add 2 to 3 tablespoons water to create a creamy yet pourable consistency. Set aside.

Make the Bowl
1. Preheat the oven to 425ºF (220ºC). Line a baking sheet with parchment paper.
2. Arrange the sweet potato on the prepared baking sheet and drizzle with the olive oil. Toss. Roast for 10 to 15 minutes, stirring once, until tender and browned.
3. In each of 2 bowls, arrange ½ cup of chickpeas, 1 cup of kale, and half of the cooked sweet potato. Drizzle with half the creamy tahini sauce and serve.

Per Serving
calories: 322 | fat: 14g | protein: 17g | carbs: 36g | sugars: 7g | fiber: 8g | sodium: 305mg

Whole-Wheat Linguine with Kale Pesto

Prep time: 10 minutes | Cook time: 20 minutes | Serves 6

½ cup shredded kale
½ cup fresh basil
½ cup sun-dried tomatoes
¼ cup chopped almonds

2 tablespoons extra-virgin olive oil
8 ounces (227 g) dry whole-wheat linguine
½ cup grated Parmesan cheese

1. Place the kale, basil, sun-dried tomatoes, almonds, and olive oil in a food processor or blender, and pulse until a chunky paste forms, about 2 minutes. Scoop the pesto into a bowl and set it aside.
2. Place a large pot filled with water on high heat and bring to a boil.
3. Cook the pasta al dente, according to the package directions.
4. Drain the pasta and toss it with the pesto and the Parmesan cheese.
5. Serve immediately.

Per Serving

calories: 217 | fat: 10g | protein: 9g | carbs: 25g | sugars: 2g | fiber: 1g | sodium: 194mg

Farro Bowl

Prep time: 5 minutes | Cook time: 25 minutes | Serves 4

3 cups water
1 cup uncooked farro
1 tablespoon extra-virgin olive oil
1 teaspoon ground cumin
½ teaspoon salt
½ teaspoon freshly

ground black pepper
4 hard-boiled eggs, sliced
1 avocado, sliced
⅓ cup plain low-fat Greek yogurt
4 lemon wedges

1. In a medium saucepan, bring the water to a boil over high heat.
2. Pour the farro into the boiling water, and stir to submerge the grains. Reduce the heat to medium and cook for 20 minutes. Drain and set aside.
3. Heat a medium skillet over medium-low heat. When hot, pour in the oil, then add the cooked farro, cumin, salt, and pepper. Cook for 3 to 5 minutes, stirring occasionally.
4. Divide the farro into four equal portions, and top each with one-quarter of the eggs, avocado, and yogurt. Add a squeeze of lemon over the top of each portion.

Per Serving

calories: 332 | fat: 16g | protein: 15g | carbs: 32g | sugars: 2g | fiber: 8g | sodium: 359mg

Parmesan Cups with White Beans

Prep time: 10 minutes | Cook time: 5 minutes | Serves 4

1 cup grated Parmesan cheese, divided
1 (15-ounce / 425-g) can low-sodium white beans, drained and rinsed
1 cucumber, peeled and finely diced
½ cup finely diced red onion
¼ cup thinly sliced

fresh basil
1 garlic clove, minced
½ jalapeño pepper, diced
1 tablespoon extra-virgin olive oil
1 tablespoon balsamic vinegar
¼ teaspoon salt
Freshly ground black pepper, to taste

1. Heat a medium nonstick skillet over medium heat. Sprinkle 2 tablespoons of cheese in a thin circle in the center of the pan, flattening it with a spatula.
2. When the cheese melts, use a spatula to flip the cheese and lightly brown the other side.
3. Remove the cheese "pancake" from the pan and place into the cup of a muffin tin, bending it gently with your hands to fit in the muffin cup.
4. Repeat with the remaining cheese until you have 8 cups.
5. In a mixing bowl, combine the beans, cucumber, onion, basil, garlic, jalapeño, olive oil, and vinegar, and season with the salt and pepper.
6. Fill each cup with the bean mixture just before serving.

Per Serving

calories: 259 | fat: 12g | protein: 15g | carbs: 24g | sugars: 4g | fiber: 8g | sodium: 551mg

Coconut Quinoa

Prep time: 15 minutes | Cook time: 25 minutes | Serves 4

2 teaspoons extra-virgin olive oil
1 sweet onion, chopped
1 tablespoon grated fresh ginger
2 teaspoons minced garlic

1 cup low-sodium chicken broth
1 cup coconut milk
1 cup quinoa, well rinsed and drained
Sea salt, to taste
¼ cup shredded, unsweetened coconut

1. Place a large saucepan over medium-high heat and add the oil.
2. Sauté the onion, ginger, and garlic until softened, about 3 minutes.
3. Add the chicken broth, coconut milk, and quinoa.
4. Bring the mixture to a boil, then reduce the heat to low and cover. Simmer the quinoa, stirring occasionally, until the quinoa is tender and most of the liquid has been absorbed, about 20 minutes.
5. Season the quinoa with salt, and serve topped with the coconut.

Per Serving
calories: 354 | fat: 21g | protein: 9g | carbs: 35g | sugars: 4g | fiber: 6g | sodium: 32mg

Faux Conch Fritters

Prep time: 15 minutes | Cook time: 20 minutes | Serves 4

4 medium egg whites
½ cup fat-free milk
1 cup chickpea crumbs
¼ teaspoon freshly ground black pepper
½ teaspoon ground cumin
3 cups frozen chopped scallops, thawed

1 small onion, finely chopped
1 small green bell pepper, finely chopped
2 celery stalks, finely chopped
2 garlic cloves, minced
Juice of 2 limes

1. Preheat the oven to 350ºF (180ºC).
2. In a large bowl, combine the egg whites, milk, and chickpea crumbs.
3. Add the black pepper and cumin and mix well.
4. Add the scallops, onion, bell pepper, celery, and garlic.

5. Form golf ball-size patties and place on a rimmed baking sheet 1 inch apart.
6. Transfer the baking sheet to the oven and cook for 5 to 7 minutes, or until golden brown.
7. Flip the patties, return to the oven, and bake for 5 to 7 minutes, or until golden brown.
8. Top with the lime juice, and serve.

Per Serving
calories: 337 | fat: 0g | protein: 50g | carbs: 24g | sugars: 4g | fiber: 6g | sodium: 464mg

Curried Black-Eyed Peas

Prep time: 15 minutes | Cook time: 25 minutes | Serves 12

1 pound (454 g) dried black-eyed peas, rinsed and drained
4 cups vegetable broth
1 cup coconut water
1 cup chopped onion
4 large carrots, coarsely chopped
1½ tablespoons curry powder

1 tablespoon minced garlic
1 teaspoon peeled and minced fresh ginger
1 tablespoon extra-virgin olive oil
Kosher salt, to taste (optional)
Lime wedges, for serving

1. In the electric pressure cooker, combine the black-eyed peas, broth, coconut water, onion, carrots, curry powder, garlic, and ginger. Drizzle the olive oil over the top.
2. Close and lock the lid of the pressure cooker. Set the valve to sealing.
3. Cook on high pressure for 25 minutes.
4. When the cooking is complete, hit Cancel and allow the pressure to release naturally for 10 minutes, then quick release any remaining pressure.
5. Once the pin drops, unlock and remove the lid.
6. Season with salt (if using) and squeeze some fresh lime juice on each serving.

Per Serving (½ cup)
calories: 112 | fat: 3g | protein: 10g | carbs: 31g | sugars: 6g | fiber: 6g | sodium: 670mg

Creamy Mac and Cheese

Prep time: 10 minutes | Cook time: 25 minutes | Serves 6

1 cup fat-free evaporated milk
½ cup skim milk
½ cup low-fat cottage cheese
½ cup low-fat Cheddar cheese
1 teaspoon nutmeg
Pinch cayenne pepper
Sea salt and freshly ground black pepper, to taste
6 cups cooked whole-wheat elbow macaroni
2 tablespoons grated Parmesan cheese

1. Preheat the oven to 350ºF (180ºC).
2. Place a large saucepan over low heat and add the evaporated milk and skim milk.
3. Heat the evaporated milk and skim milk until steaming, then stir in the cottage cheese and Cheddar, stirring until they melt.
4. Stir in the nutmeg and cayenne.
5. Season the sauce with salt and black pepper and remove from the heat.
6. Stir the cooked pasta into the sauce, then spoon the mac and cheese into a large casserole dish.
7. Sprinkle the top with the Parmesan cheese, and bake until it is bubbly and lightly browned, about 20 minutes.

Per Serving
calories: 246 | fat: 2g | protein: 16g | carbs: 44g | sugars: 7g | fiber: 4g | sodium: 187mg

Tomato Baked Beans

Prep time: 10 minutes | Cook time: 25 minutes | Serves 8

1 teaspoon extra-virgin olive oil
½ sweet onion, chopped
2 teaspoons minced garlic
2 sweet potatoes, peeled and diced
1 (28-ounce / 794-g) can low-sodium diced tomatoes
¼ cup sodium-free tomato paste
2 tablespoons granulated sweetener
2 tablespoons hot sauce
1 tablespoon Dijon mustard
3 (15-ounce / 425-g) cans sodium-free navy or white beans, drained
1 tablespoon chopped fresh oregano

1. Place a large saucepan over medium-high heat and add the oil.
2. Sauté the onion and garlic until translucent, about 3 minutes.
3. Stir in the sweet potatoes, diced tomatoes, tomato paste, sweetener, hot sauce, and mustard and bring to a boil.
4. Reduce the heat and simmer the tomato sauce for 10 minutes.
5. Stir in the beans and simmer for 10 minutes more.
6. Stir in the oregano and serve.

Per Serving
calories: 255 | fat: 2g | protein: 15g | carbs: 48g | sugars: 8g | fiber: 12g | sodium: 149mg

Whole-Wheat Couscous with Pecans

Prep time: 10 minutes | Cook time: 5 minutes | Serves 6

Dressing:
¼ cup extra-virgin olive oil
2 tablespoons balsamic vinegar
1 teaspoon honey
Sea salt and freshly ground black pepper, to taste

Couscous:
1¼ cups whole-wheat couscous
Pinch sea salt
1 teaspoon butter
2 cups boiling water
1 scallion, white and green parts, chopped
½ cup chopped pecans
2 tablespoons chopped fresh parsley

Make the Dressing
Whisk together the oil, vinegar, and honey.
1. Season with salt and pepper and set it aside.

Make the Couscous
2. Put the couscous, salt, and butter in a large heat-proof bowl and pour the boiling water on top. Stir and cover the bowl. Let it sit for 5 minutes. Uncover and fluff the couscous with a fork.
3. Stir in the dressing, scallion, pecans, and parsley.
4. Serve warm.

Per Serving
calories: 251 | fat: 13g | protein: 5g | carbs: 30g | sugars: 1g | fiber: 2g | sodium: 76mg

Baked Egg Skillet with Avocado

Prep time: 5 minutes | Cook time: 25 minutes | Serves 4

2 tablespoons extra-virgin olive oil
1 red onion, chopped
1 green bell pepper, seeded and chopped
1 sweet potato, cut into ½-inch pieces
1 teaspoon chili powder
½ teaspoon sea salt
4 large eggs
½ cup shredded pepper Jack cheese
1 avocado, cut into cubes

1. Preheat the oven to 350ºF (180ºC).
2. In a large, ovenproof skillet over medium-high heat, heat the olive oil until it shimmers. Add the onion, bell pepper, sweet potato, chili powder, and salt, and cook, stirring occasionally, until the vegetables start to brown, about 10 minutes.
3. Remove from heat. Arrange the vegetables in the pan to form 4 wells. Crack an egg into each well. Sprinkle the cheese on the vegetables, around the edges of the eggs.
4. Bake until the eggs set, about 10 minutes.
5. Top with avocado before serving.

Per Serving
calories: 284 | fat: 21g | protein: 12g | carbs: 16g | sugars: 3g | fiber: 5g | sodium: 264mg

Vegetable Kale Lasagna

Prep time: 20 minutes | Cook time: 1 hour | Serves 6

1 tablespoon extra-virgin olive oil
1 sweet onion, chopped
2 teaspoons minced garlic
½ small eggplant, chopped
1 green zucchini, chopped
1 yellow zucchini, chopped
1 red bell pepper, seeded and diced
1 (28-ounce / 794-g) can sodium-free diced tomatoes
1 cup shredded kale
1 tablespoon chopped fresh basil
2 teaspoons chopped fresh oregano
Pinch red pepper flakes
12 whole-wheat lasagna noodles, cooked according to package instructions
½ cup grated Parmesan cheese
½ cup fat-free Mozzarella cheese

1. Preheat the oven to 400ºF (205ºC).
2. Place a large saucepan over medium-high heat and add the olive oil.
3. Sauté the onion and garlic until softened and translucent, about 3 minutes.
4. Stir in the eggplant, green and yellow zucchini, bell pepper, tomatoes, and kale.
5. Bring the sauce to a boil, then reduce the heat to low and simmer for 15 minutes.
6. Remove the sauce from the heat and stir in the basil, oregano, and red pepper flakes.
7. Scoop one quarter of the sauce into a 9-by-13-inch rectangular baking pan. Top with 4 noodles. Repeat with a layer of sauce, noodles, sauce, noodles, and the final layer of sauce on top. Sprinkle with the Parmesan cheese and Mozzarella.
8. Bake the lasagna until it's bubbly and hot, about 45 minutes.
9. Cool for 10 minutes and serve.

Per Serving
calories: 313 | fat: 8g | protein: 16g | carbs: 48g | sugars: 7g | fiber: 5g | sodium: 165mg

Green Lentils with Olives and Vegetables

Prep time: 15 minutes | Cook time: 0 minutes | Serves 4

3 tablespoons extra-virgin olive oil
2 tablespoons balsamic vinegar
2 teaspoons chopped fresh basil
1 teaspoon minced garlic
Sea salt and freshly ground black pepper, to taste
2 (15-ounce / 425-g) cans sodium-free green lentils, rinsed and drained
½ English cucumber, diced
2 tomatoes, diced
½ cup halved Kalamata olives
¼ cup chopped fresh chives
2 tablespoons pine nuts

1. Whisk together the olive oil, vinegar, basil, and garlic in a medium bowl. Season with salt and pepper.
2. Stir in the lentils, cucumber, tomatoes, olives, and chives.
3. Top with the pine nuts, and serve.

Per Serving
calories: 399 | fat: 15g | protein: 20g | carbs: 49g | sugars: 7g | fiber: 19g | sodium: 438mg

Chickpea Lentil Curry

Prep time: 10 minutes | Cook time: 25 minutes | Serves 6

1 tablespoon extra-virgin olive oil
1 sweet onion, chopped
1 tablespoon grated fresh ginger
1 teaspoon minced garlic
2 tablespoons red curry paste
1 teaspoon ground cumin
½ teaspoon turmeric
Pinch cayenne pepper
1 (28-ounce / 794-g) can sodium-free diced tomatoes
2 cups cooked lentils
1 (15-ounce / 425-g) can water-packed chickpeas, rinsed and drained
¼ cup coconut milk
2 tablespoons chopped fresh cilantro

1. Place a large saucepan over medium-high heat and add the oil.
2. Sauté the onion, ginger, and garlic until softened, about 3 minutes.
3. Add the curry paste, cumin, turmeric, and cayenne and sauté 1 minute more.
4. Stir in the tomatoes, lentils, chickpeas, and coconut milk.
5. Bring the curry to a boil, then reduce the heat to low and simmer for 20 minutes.
6. Remove the curry from the heat and garnish with the cilantro.

Per Serving
calories: 338 | fat: 8g | protein: 18g | carbs: 50g | sugars: 9g | fiber: 20g | sodium: 22mg

Sweet Potato Fennel Bake

Prep time: 15 minutes | Cook time: 45 minutes | Serves 4

1 teaspoon butter
1 fennel bulb, trimmed and thinly sliced
2 sweet potatoes, peeled and thinly sliced
Freshly ground black pepper, to taste
½ teaspoon ground cinnamon
¼ teaspoon ground nutmeg
1 cup low-sodium vegetable broth

1. Preheat the oven to 375ºF (190ºC).
2. Lightly butter a 9-by-11-inch baking dish.
3. Arrange half the fennel in the bottom of the dish and top with half the sweet potatoes.
4. Season the potatoes with black pepper. Sprinkle half the cinnamon and nutmeg on the potatoes.
5. Repeat the layering to use up all the fennel, sweet potatoes, cinnamon, and nutmeg.
6. Pour in the vegetable broth and cover the dish with aluminum foil.
7. Bake until the vegetables are very tender, about 45 minutes.
8. Serve immediately.

Per Serving
calories: 153 | fat: 2g | protein: 3g | carbs: 33g | sugars: 1g | fiber: 7g | sodium: 178mg

Barley Squash Risotto

Prep time: 10 minutes | Cook time: 15 minutes | Serves 6

1 teaspoon extra-virgin olive oil
½ sweet onion, finely chopped
1 teaspoon minced garlic
2 cups cooked barley
2 cups chopped kale
2 cups cooked butternut squash, cut into ½-inch cubes
2 tablespoons chopped pistachios
1 tablespoon chopped fresh thyme
Sea salt, to taste

1. Place a large skillet over medium heat and add the oil.
2. Sauté the onion and garlic until softened and translucent, about 3 minutes.
3. Add the barley and kale, and stir until the grains are heated through and the greens are wilted, about 7 minutes.
4. Stir in the squash, pistachios, and thyme.
5. Cook until the dish is hot, about 4 minutes, and season with salt.

Per Serving
calories: 159 | fat: 2g | protein: 5g | carbs: 32g | sugars: 2g | fiber: 7g | sodium: 62mg

Mushroom Cutlets with Creamy Sauce

Prep time: 15 minutes | Cook time: 20 minutes | Serves 4

Sauce:

1 tablespoon extra-virgin olive oil
2 tablespoons whole-wheat flour
1½ cups unsweetened plain almond milk

¼ teaspoon salt
Dash Worcestershire sauce
Pinch cayenne pepper
¼ cup shredded Cheddar cheese

Cutlets:

2 eggs
2 cups chopped mushrooms
1 cup quick oats
2 scallions, both white and green parts, chopped

¼ cup shredded Cheddar cheese
½ teaspoon salt
¼ teaspoon freshly ground black pepper
1 tablespoon extra-virgin olive oil

Make the Sauce

1. In a medium saucepan, heat the oil over medium heat. Add the flour and stir constantly for about 2 minutes until browned.
2. Slowly whisk in the almond milk and bring to a boil. Reduce the heat to low and simmer for 6 to 8 minutes until the sauce thickens.
3. Season with the salt, Worcestershire sauce, and cayenne. Add the cheese and stir until melted. Turn off the heat and cover to keep warm while you make the cutlets.

Make the Cutlets

1. In a large mixing bowl, beat the eggs. Add the mushrooms, oats, scallions, cheese, salt, and pepper. Stir to combine.
2. Using your hands, form the mixture into 8 patties, each about ½ inch thick.
3. In a large skillet, heat the oil over medium-high heat. Cook the patties, in batches if necessary, for 3 minutes per side until crisp and brown.
4. Serve the cutlets warm with sauce drizzled over the top.

Per Serving

calories: 261 | fat: 17g | protein: 11g | carbs: 18g | sugars: 2g | fiber: 3g | sodium: 559mg

Falafel with Creamy Garlic-Yogurt Sauce

Prep time: 15 minutes | Cook time: 10 minutes | Serves 4

Sauce:

¾ cup plain nonfat Greek yogurt
3 garlic cloves, minced

Juice of 1 lemon
1 tablespoon extra-virgin olive oil
¼ teaspoon salt

Falafel:

1 (15-ounce / 425-g) can low-sodium chickpeas, drained and rinsed
2 garlic cloves, roughly chopped
2 tablespoons whole-wheat flour
2 tablespoons chopped fresh parsley

½ teaspoon ground cumin
¼ teaspoon salt
2 teaspoons canola oil, divided
8 large lettuce leaves, chopped
1 cucumber, chopped
1 tomato, diced

Make the Sauce

1. In a small bowl, combine the yogurt, garlic, lemon juice, olive oil, and salt, and mix well. Cover and refrigerate until ready to serve.

Make the Falafel

1. In a food processor or blender, combine the chickpeas and garlic, and pulse until chopped well but not creamy. Add the flour, parsley, cumin, and salt. Pulse several more times until incorporated.
2. Using your hands, form the mixture into balls, using about 1 tablespoon of mixture for each ball.
3. In a medium skillet, heat 1 teaspoon of canola oil over medium-high heat. Working in batches, add the falafel to the skillet, cooking on each side for 2 to 3 minutes until browned and crisp. Remove the falafel from the skillet, and repeat with the remaining oil and falafel until all are cooked.
4. Divide the lettuce, cucumber, and tomato among 4 plates.
5. Top each plate with 2 falafel and 2 tablespoons of sauce. Serve immediately.

Per Serving

calories: 219 | fat: 8g | protein: 12g | carbs: 27g | sugars: 6g | fiber: 7g | sodium: 462mg

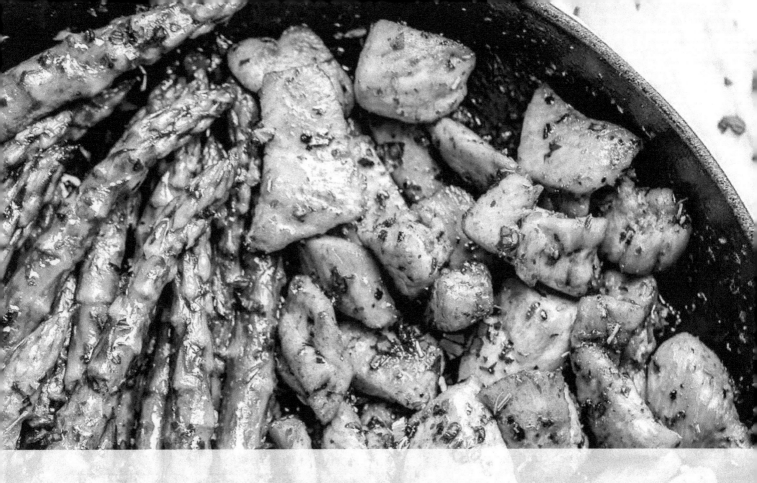
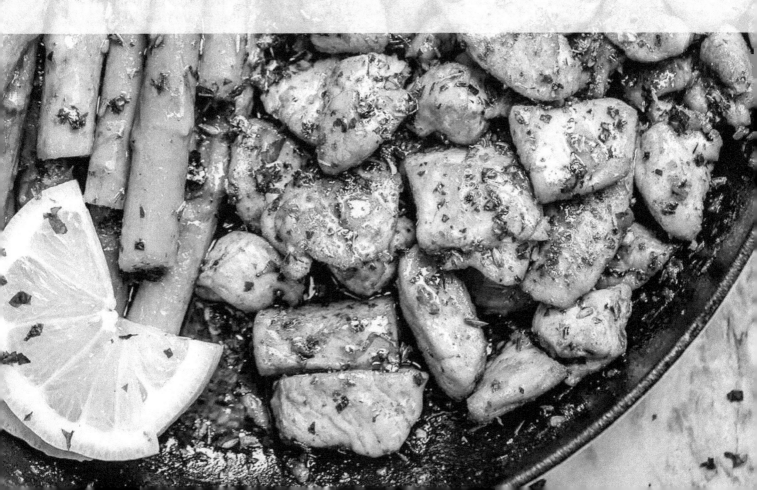

Chapter 6 Poultry

Baked Coconut Chicken Tenders

Prep time: 10 minutes | Cook time: 20 minutes | Serves 6

4 chicken breasts, each cut lengthwise into 3 strips
½ teaspoon salt
¼ teaspoon freshly ground black pepper
½ cup coconut flour

2 eggs, beaten
2 tablespoons unsweetened plain almond milk
1 cup unsweetened coconut flakes

1. Preheat the oven to 400ºF (205ºC). Line a baking sheet with parchment paper.
2. Season the chicken pieces with the salt and pepper.
3. Place the coconut flour in a small bowl. In another bowl, mix the eggs with the almond milk. Spread the coconut flakes on a plate.
4. One by one, roll the chicken pieces in the flour, then dip the floured chicken in the egg mixture and shake off any excess. Roll in the coconut flakes and transfer to the prepared baking sheet.
5. Bake for 15 to 20 minutes, flipping once halfway through, until cooked through and browned.

Per Serving

calories: 216 | fat: 13g | protein: 20g | carbs: 9g | sugars: 2g | fiber: 6g | sodium: 346mg

Honey Mustard Chicken Lettuce Wraps

Prep time: 10 minutes | Cook time: 0 minutes | Serves 4

8 romaine lettuce leaves
1½ cups shredded rotisserie chicken
1 avocado, sliced
2 hard-boiled eggs,

sliced
1 medium tomato, sliced
4 teaspoons honey mustard

1. Top each lettuce leaf with one-eighth of the chicken, avocado, eggs, and tomato.
2. Drizzle the honey mustard over the filling, and working from the edge closest to you, roll up each lettuce leaf to make the wraps.

Per Serving

calories: 227 | fat: 11g | protein:24g | carbs: 8g | sugars: 3g | fiber: 4g | sodium: 159mg

Open-Faced Greek Chicken Sandwiches

Prep time: 10 minutes | Cook time: 0 minutes | Serves 3

3 tablespoons red pepper hummus
3 slices 100% whole-wheat bread, toasted
¾ cup cucumber slices
3 cups arugula or

baby kale
¼ cup sliced red onion
1 cup shredded rotisserie chicken
Oregano, for garnish (optional)

1. Spread 1 tablespoon of hummus on each slice of toasted bread.
2. Layer one-third of the cucumber, arugula, onion, and chicken on each slice of bread. Garnish with oregano (if using).

Per Serving

calories: 288 | fat: 6g | protein: 23g | carbs: 25g | sugars: 4g | fiber: 4g | sodium: 331mg

Teriyaki Meatballs

Prep time: 20 minutes | Cook time: 20 minutes | Serves 6

1 pound (454 g) lean ground turkey
¼ cup finely chopped scallions, both white and green parts
1 egg
2 garlic cloves, minced
1 teaspoon grated

fresh ginger
2 tablespoons reduced-sodium tamari or gluten-free soy sauce
1 tablespoon honey
2 teaspoons mirin
1 teaspoon toasted sesame oil

1. Preheat the oven to 400ºF (205ºC). Line a baking sheet with parchment paper.
2. In a large mixing bowl, combine the turkey, scallions, egg, garlic, ginger, tamari, honey, mirin, and sesame oil. Mix well.
3. Using your hands, form the meat mixture into balls about the size of a tablespoon. Arrange on the prepared baking sheet.
4. Bake for 10 minutes, flip with a spatula, and continue baking for an additional 10 minutes until the meatballs are cooked through.

Per Serving

calories: 153 | fat: 8g | protein: 16g | carbs: 5g | sugars: 4g | fiber: 0g | sodium: 270mg

Chicken Caesar Salad

Prep time: 10 minutes | Cook time: 15 minutes | Serves 2

1 garlic clove
½ teaspoon anchovy paste
Juice of ½ lemon
2 tablespoons extra-virgin olive oil
1 (8-ounce / 227-g) boneless, skinless chicken breast
¼ teaspoon salt
Freshly ground black pepper, to taste
2 romaine lettuce hearts, cored and chopped
1 red bell pepper, seeded and cut into thin strips
¼ cup grated Parmesan cheese

1. Preheat the broiler to high.
2. In a blender jar, combine the garlic, anchovy paste, lemon juice, and olive oil. Process until smooth and set aside.
3. Cut the chicken breast lengthwise into two even cutlets of similar thickness. Season the chicken with the salt and pepper, and place on a baking sheet.
4. Broil the chicken for 5 to 7 minutes on each side until cooked through and browned. Cut into thin strips.
5. In a medium mixing bowl, toss the lettuce, bell pepper, and cheese. Add the dressing and toss to coat. Divide the salad between 2 plates and top with the chicken.

Per Serving

calories: 292 | fat: 18g | protein: 28g | carbs: 6g | sugars: 3g | fiber: 2g | sodium: 706mg

Savory Rubbed Roast Chicken

Prep time: 10 minutes | Cook time: 35 minutes | Serves 6

1 teaspoon ground paprika
1 teaspoon garlic powder
½ teaspoon ground coriander
½ teaspoon ground cumin
½ teaspoon salt
¼ teaspoon ground cayenne pepper
6 chicken legs
1 teaspoon extra-virgin olive oil

1. Preheat the oven to 400ºF (205ºC).
2. In a small bowl, combine the paprika, garlic powder, coriander, cumin, salt, and cayenne pepper. Rub the chicken legs all over with the spices.

3. In an ovenproof skillet, heat the oil over medium heat. Sear the chicken for 8 to 10 minutes on each side until the skin browns and becomes crisp.
4. Transfer the skillet to the oven and continue to cook for 10 to 15 minutes until the chicken is cooked through and its juices run clear.

Per Serving

calories: 276 | fat: 16g | protein: 30g | carbs: 1g | sugars: 0g | fiber: 0g | sodium: 256mg

Turkey Chili

Prep time: 15 minutes | Cook time: 30 minutes | Serves 6

1 tablespoon extra-virgin olive oil
1 pound (454 g) lean ground turkey
1 large onion, diced
3 garlic cloves, minced
1 red bell pepper, seeded and diced
1 cup chopped celery
2 tablespoons chili powder
1 tablespoon ground cumin
1 (28-ounce / 794-g) can reduced-salt diced tomatoes
1 (15-ounce / 425-g) can low-sodium kidney beans, drained and rinsed
2 cups low-sodium chicken broth
½ teaspoon salt
Shredded Cheddar cheese, for serving (optional)

1. In a large pot, heat the oil over medium heat. Add the turkey, onion, and garlic, and cook, stirring regularly, until the turkey is cooked through.
2. Add the bell pepper, celery, chili powder, and cumin. Stir well and continue to cook for 1 minute.
3. Add the tomatoes with their liquid, kidney beans, and chicken broth. Bring to a boil, reduce the heat to low, and simmer for 20 minutes.
4. Season with the salt and serve topped with cheese (if using).

Per Serving

calories: 276 | fat: 10g | protein: 23g | carbs: 27g | sugars: 7g | fiber: 8g | sodium: 556mg

Saffron Chicken

Prep time: 10 minutes | Cook time: 10 minutes | Serves 4

Pinch saffron (3 or 4 threads)
½ cup plain nonfat yogurt
2 tablespoons water
½ onion, chopped
3 garlic cloves, minced
2 tablespoons

chopped fresh cilantro
Juice of ½ lemon
½ teaspoon salt
1 pound (454 g) boneless, skinless chicken breasts, cut into 2-inch strips
1 tablespoon extra-virgin olive oil

1. In a blender jar, combine the saffron, yogurt, water, onion, garlic, cilantro, lemon juice, and salt. Pulse to blend.
2. In a large mixing bowl, combine the chicken and the yogurt sauce, and stir to coat. Cover and refrigerate for at least 1 hour or up to overnight.
3. In a large skillet, heat the oil over medium heat. Add the chicken pieces, shaking off any excess marinade. Discard the marinade. Cook the chicken pieces on each side for 5 minutes, flipping once, until cooked through and golden brown.

Per Serving
calories: 155 | fat: 5g | protein: 26g | carbs: 3g | sugars: 1g | fiber: 0g | sodium: 501mg

Sesame Chicken Soba Noodles

Prep time: 10 minutes | Cook time: 15 minutes | Serves 6

8 ounces (227 g) soba noodles
2 boneless, skinless chicken breasts, halved lengthwise
¼ cup tahini
2 tablespoons rice vinegar
1 tablespoon reduced-sodium gluten-free soy sauce or tamari

1 teaspoon toasted sesame oil
1 (1-inch) piece fresh ginger, finely grated
1/3 cup water
1 large cucumber, seeded and diced
1 scallions bunch, green parts only, cut into 1-inch segments
1 tablespoon sesame seeds

1. Preheat the broiler to high.
2. Bring a large pot of water to a boil. Add the noodles and cook until tender, according to the package directions. Drain and rinse the noodles in cool water.
3. On a baking sheet, arrange the chicken in a single layer. Broil for 5 to 7 minutes on each side, depending on the thickness, until the chicken is cooked through and its juices run clear. Use two forks to shred the chicken.
4. In a small bowl, combine the tahini, rice vinegar, soy sauce, sesame oil, ginger, and water. Whisk to combine.
5. In a large bowl, toss the shredded chicken, noodles, cucumber, and scallions. Pour the tahini sauce over the noodles and toss to combine. Served sprinkled with the sesame seeds.

Per Serving
calories: 251 | fat: 8g | protein: 16g | carbs: 35g | sugars: 2g | fiber: 2g | sodium: 482mg

Smothered Dijon Chicken

Prep time: 10 minutes | Cook time: 30 minutes | Serves 4

¾ cup low-fat buttermilk
2 tablespoons Dijon mustard
3 garlic cloves, minced
1 tablespoon dried dill
1 teaspoon mustard

seeds
2 boneless, skinless chicken breasts
2 large carrots, peeled and halved
1 medium onion, quartered

1. Preheat the oven to 375ºF (190ºC).
2. In a medium bowl, combine the buttermilk, mustard, garlic, dill, and mustard seeds. Mix well.
3. Add the chicken, carrots, and onion, coating them thoroughly with the buttermilk mixture. Set aside to marinate for at least 15 minutes.
4. Place the chicken, carrots, and onions on a rimmed baking sheet. Discard the remaining buttermilk mixture.
5. Transfer the baking sheet to the oven, and bake for 30 minutes, or until the vegetables are tender, and the chicken is cooked through and its juices run clear. Serve warm and enjoy.

Per Serving
calories: 119 | fat: 2g | protein: 16g | carbs: 10g | sugars: 5g | fiber: 2g | sodium: 202mg

Chicken Salad Sandwiches

Prep time: 10 minutes | Cook time: 10 minutes | Serves 4

Avocado oil cooking spray
2 (4-ounce / 113-g) boneless, skinless chicken breasts
⅛ teaspoon freshly ground black pepper
1½ tablespoons plain low-fat Greek yogurt
¼ cup halved purple seedless grapes
¼ cup chopped pecans
2 tablespoons chopped celery
4 sandwich thins, 100% whole-wheat

1. Heat a small skillet over medium-low heat. When hot, coat the cooking surface with cooking spray.
2. Season the chicken with the pepper. Place the chicken in the skillet and cook for 6 minutes. Flip and cook for 3 to 5 minutes more, or until cooked through.
3. Remove the chicken from the skillet and let cool for 5 minutes.
4. Chop or shred the chicken.
5. Combine the chicken, yogurt, grapes, pecans, and celery.
6. Cut the sandwich thins in half, so there is a top and bottom.
7. Divide the chicken salad into four equal portions, spoon one portion on each of the bottom halves of the sandwich thins, and cover with the top halves.

Per Serving
calories: 250 | fat: 8g | protein: 23g | carbs: 24g | sugars: 4g | fiber: 6g | sodium: 209mg

Caesar Chicken Sandwiches

Prep time: 5 minutes | Cook time: 0 minutes | Serves 4

Dressing:
4 tablespoons plain low-fat Greek yogurt
4 teaspoons Dijon mustard
4 teaspoons freshly squeezed lemon juice
4 teaspoons shredded Parmesan cheese
¼ teaspoon freshly ground black pepper
⅛ teaspoon garlic powder
Sandwiches:
2 cups shredded rotisserie chicken
1½ cups chopped romaine lettuce
12 cherry tomatoes, halved
4 sandwich thins, 100% whole-wheat
¼ cup thinly sliced red onion (optional)

Make the Dressing
1. In a small bowl, whisk together the yogurt, mustard, lemon juice, Parmesan cheese, black pepper, and garlic powder.

Make the Sandwiches
1. In a large bowl, combine the chicken, lettuce, and tomatoes. Add the dressing and stir until evenly coated. Divide the filling into four equal portions.
2. Slice the sandwich thins so there is a top and bottom half for each. Put one portion of filling on each of the bottom halves and cover with the top halves.

Per Serving
calories: 242 | fat: 5g | protein: 28g | carbs: 25g | sugars: 4g | fiber: 8g | sodium: 359mg

Chicken and Onion Grilled Cheese

Prep time: 10 minutes | Cook time: 15 minutes | Serves 4

1 small yellow onion
Avocado oil cooking spray
2 cups shredded rotisserie chicken
1½ tablespoons
unsalted butter
4 slices 100% whole-wheat bread
3 slices provolone or Swiss cheese
2 cups fresh spinach

1. Cut the onion into ½-inch rounds. Leave them intact; do not separate.
2. Heat a medium or large skillet over medium-low heat. When hot, coat the cooking surface with cooking spray. Place the onions in the skillet. Cover and cook for 7 to 10 minutes, or until the onions are translucent. Remove from the skillet.
3. Meanwhile, shred the chicken, and butter one side of each slice of bread. Tear each slice of cheese into 3 strips.
4. Place 2 or 3 strips of cheese on the nonbuttered side of each piece of bread, then place the buttered side down on the skillet.
5. Layer one-quarter of the onion, spinach, and shredded chicken on top of each slice of bread.
6. Toast for 2 to 3 minutes over medium-low heat.

Per Serving
calories: 318 | fat: 13g | protein: 27g | carbs: 23g | sugars: 3g | fiber: 4g | sodium: 496mg

One-Pan Chicken Dinner

Prep time: 5 minutes | Cook time: 35 minutes | Serves 4

3 tablespoons extra-virgin olive oil
1 tablespoon red wine vinegar or apple cider vinegar
¼ teaspoon garlic powder
3 tablespoons Italian seasoning
4 (4-ounce / 113-g) boneless, skinless chicken breasts
2 cups cubed sweet potatoes
20 Brussels sprouts, halved lengthwise

1. Preheat the oven to 400ºF (205ºC).
2. In a large bowl, whisk together the oil, vinegar, garlic powder, and Italian seasoning.
3. Add the chicken, sweet potatoes, and Brussels sprouts, and coat thoroughly with the marinade.
4. Remove the ingredients from the marinade and arrange them on a baking sheet in a single layer. Roast for 15 minutes.
5. Remove the baking sheet from the oven, flip the chicken over, and bake for another 15 to 20 minutes.

Per Serving
calories: 342 | fat: 16g | protein: 30g | carbs: 23g | sugars: 8g | fiber: 9g | sodium: 186mg

Greek Chicken Stuffed Peppers

Prep time: 5 minutes | Cook time: 30 minutes | Serves 4

2 large red bell peppers
2 teaspoons extra-virgin olive oil, divided
½ cup uncooked brown rice or quinoa
4 (4-ounce / 113-g) boneless, skinless chicken breasts
¼ teaspoon garlic powder
¼ teaspoon onion powder
⅛ teaspoon dried thyme
½ teaspoon dried oregano
½ cup crumbled feta

1. Cut the bell peppers in half and remove the seeds.
2. In a large skillet, heat 1 teaspoon of olive oil over low heat. When hot, place the bell pepper halves cut-side up in the skillet. Cover and cook for 20 minutes.
3. Cook the rice according to the package instructions.
4. Meanwhile, cut the chicken into 1-inch pieces.
5. In a medium skillet, heat the remaining 1 teaspoon of olive oil over medium-low heat. When hot, add the chicken.
6. Season the chicken with the garlic powder, onion powder, thyme, and oregano.
7. Cook for 5 minutes, stirring occasionally, until cooked through.
8. In a large bowl, combine the cooked rice and chicken. Scoop one-quarter of the chicken and rice mixture into each pepper half, cover, and cook for 10 minutes over low heat.
9. Top each pepper half with 2 tablespoons of crumbled feta.

Per Serving
calories: 288 | fat: 10g | protein: 32g | carbs: 20g | sugars: 4g | fiber: 4g | sodium: 267mg

Baked Turkey Spaghetti

Prep time: 5 minutes | Cook time: 20 minutes | Serves 4

1 (10-ounce / 283-g) package zucchini noodles
2 tablespoons extra-virgin olive oil, divided
1 pound (454 g) 93% lean ground turkey
½ teaspoon dried oregano
2 cups low-sodium spaghetti sauce
½ cup shredded sharp Cheddar cheese

1. Pat zucchini noodles dry between two paper towels.
2. In an oven-safe medium skillet, heat 1 tablespoon of olive oil over medium heat. When hot, add the zucchini noodles. Cook for 3 minutes, stirring halfway through.
3. Add the remaining 1 tablespoon of oil, ground turkey, and oregano. Cook for 7 to 10 minutes, stirring and breaking apart, as needed.
4. Add the spaghetti sauce to the skillet and stir.
5. If your broiler is in the top of your oven, place the oven rack in the center position. Set the broiler on high.
6. Top the mixture with the cheese, and broil for 5 minutes or until the cheese is bubbly.

Per Serving
calories: 335 | fat: 21g | protein: 28g | carbs: 12g | sugars: 4g | fiber: 3g | sodium: 216mg

Taco Stuffed Sweet Potatoes

Prep time: 5 minutes | Cook time: 15 minutes | Serves 4

4 medium sweet potatoes
2 tablespoons extra-virgin olive oil
1 pound (454 g) 93% lean ground turkey
2 teaspoons ground
cumin
1 teaspoon chili powder
½ teaspoon salt
½ teaspoon freshly ground black pepper

1. Pierce the potatoes with a fork, and microwave them on the potato setting, or for 10 minutes on high power.
2. Meanwhile, heat a medium skillet over medium heat. When hot, put the oil, turkey, cumin, chili powder, salt, and pepper into the skillet, stirring and breaking apart the meat, as needed.
3. Remove the potatoes from the microwave and halve them lengthwise. Depress the centers with a spoon, and fill each half with an equal amount of cooked turkey.

Per Serving

calories: 300 | fat: 8g | protein: 30g | carbs: 27g | sugars: 4g | fiber: 5g | sodium: 426mg

Chicken Romaine Salad

Prep time: 15 minutes | Cook time: 0 minutes | Serves 4

2 cups shredded rotisserie chicken
1½ tablespoons plain low-fat Greek yogurt
⅛ teaspoon freshly ground black pepper
¼ cup halved purple
seedless grapes
8 cups chopped romaine lettuce
1 medium tomato, sliced
1 avocado, sliced

1. In a large bowl, combine the chicken, yogurt, and pepper, and mix well.
2. Stir in the grapes.
3. Divide the lettuce into four portions. Spoon one-quarter of the chicken salad onto each portion and top with a couple slices of tomato and avocado.

Per Serving

calories: 203 | fat: 10g | protein: 22g | carbs: 10g | sugars: 4g | fiber: 5g | sodium: 56mg

Turkey Divan Casserole

Prep time: 10 minutes | Cook time: 50 minutes | Serves 6

Nonstick cooking spray
3 teaspoons extra-virgin olive oil, divided
1 pound (454 g) turkey cutlets
Pinch salt
¼ teaspoon freshly ground black pepper, divided
¼ cup chopped onion
2 garlic cloves, minced
2 tablespoons whole-
wheat flour
1 cup unsweetened plain almond milk
1 cup low-sodium chicken broth
½ cup shredded Swiss cheese, divided
½ teaspoon dried thyme
4 cups chopped broccoli
¼ cup coarsely ground almonds

1. Preheat the oven to 375ºF (190ºC). Spray a baking dish with nonstick cooking spray.
2. In a skillet, heat 1 teaspoon of oil over medium heat. Season the turkey with the salt and ⅛ teaspoon of pepper. Sauté the turkey cutlets for 5 to 7 minutes on each side until cooked through. Transfer to a cutting board, cool briefly, and cut into bite-size pieces.
3. In the same pan, heat the remaining 2 teaspoons of oil over medium-high heat. Sauté the onion for 3 minutes until it begins to soften. Add the garlic and continue cooking for another minute.
4. Stir in the flour and mix well. Whisk in the almond milk, broth, and remaining ⅛ teaspoon of pepper, and continue whisking until smooth. Add ¼ cup of cheese and the thyme, and continue stirring until the cheese is melted.
5. In the prepared baking dish, arrange the broccoli on the bottom. Cover with half the sauce. Place the turkey pieces on top of the broccoli, and cover with the remaining sauce. Sprinkle with the remaining ¼ cup of cheese and the ground almonds.
6. Bake for 35 minutes until the sauce is bubbly and the top is browned.

Per Serving

calories: 207 | fat: 8g | protein: 25g | carbs: 9g | sugars: 2g | fiber: 3g | sodium: 128mg

Coconut Lime Chicken

Prep time: 5 minutes | Cook time: 15 minutes | Serves 4

1 tablespoon coconut oil
4 (4-ounce / 113-g) boneless, skinless chicken breasts
½ teaspoon salt
1 red bell pepper, cut into ¼-inch-thick slices
16 asparagus spears, bottom ends trimmed

1 cup unsweetened coconut milk
2 tablespoons freshly squeezed lime juice
½ teaspoon garlic powder
¼ teaspoon red pepper flakes
¼ cup chopped fresh cilantro

1. In a large skillet, heat the oil over medium-low heat. When hot, add the chicken.
2. Season the chicken with the salt. Cook for 5 minutes, then flip.
3. Push the chicken to the side of the skillet, and add the bell pepper and asparagus. Cook, covered, for 5 minutes.
4. Meanwhile, in a small bowl, whisk together the coconut milk, lime juice, garlic powder, and red pepper flakes.
5. Add the coconut milk mixture to the skillet, and boil over high heat for 2 to 3 minutes.
6. Top with the cilantro.

Per Serving
calories: 321 | fat: 19g | protein: 30g | carbs: 11g | sugars: 6g | fiber: 4g | sodium: 378mg

Creamy Garlic Chicken with Broccoli

Prep time: 5 minutes | Cook time: 15 minutes | Serves 4

½ cup uncooked brown rice or quinoa
4 (4-ounce / 113-g) boneless, skinless chicken breasts
¼ teaspoon salt
¼ teaspoon freshly ground black pepper

1 teaspoon garlic powder, divided
Avocado oil cooking spray
3 cups fresh or frozen broccoli florets
1 cup half-and-half

1. Cook the rice according to the package instructions.
2. Meanwhile, season both sides of the chicken breasts with the salt, pepper, and ½ teaspoon of garlic powder.

3. Heat a large skillet over medium-low heat. When hot, coat the cooking surface with cooking spray and add the chicken and broccoli in a single layer.
4. Cook for 4 minutes, then flip the chicken breasts over and cover. Cook for 5 minutes more.
5. Add the half-and-half and remaining ½ teaspoon of garlic powder to the skillet and stir. Increase the heat to high and simmer for 2 minutes.
6. Divide the rice into four equal portions. Top each portion with 1 chicken breast and one-quarter of the broccoli and cream sauce.

Per Serving
calories: 303 | fat: 10g | protein: 33g | carbs: 22g | sugars: 4g | fiber: 3g | sodium: 271mg

Peppered Chicken with Balsamic Kale

Prep time: 5 minutes | Cook time: 15 minutes | Serves 4

4 (4-ounce / 113-g) boneless, skinless chicken breasts
¼ teaspoon salt
1 tablespoon freshly ground black pepper
2 tablespoons unsalted butter
1 tablespoon extra-

virgin olive oil
8 cups stemmed and roughly chopped kale, loosely packed (about 2 bunches)
½ cup balsamic vinegar
20 cherry tomatoes, halved

1. Season both sides of the chicken breasts with the salt and pepper.
2. Heat a large skillet over medium heat. When hot, heat the butter and oil. Add the chicken and cook for 8 to 10 minutes, flipping halfway through. When cooked all the way through, remove the chicken from the skillet and set aside.
3. Increase the heat to medium-high. Put the kale in the skillet and cook for 3 minutes, stirring every minute.
4. Add the vinegar and the tomatoes and cook for another 3 to 5 minutes.
5. Divide the kale and tomato mixture into four equal portions, and top each portion with 1 chicken breast.

Per Serving
calories: 293 | fat: 11g | protein: 31g | carbs: 18g | sugars: 4g | fiber: 3g | sodium: 328mg

Ground Turkey Taco Skillet

Prep time: 10 minutes | Cook time: 20 minutes | Serves 4

3 tablespoons extra-virgin olive oil
1 pound (454 g) ground turkey
1 onion, chopped
1 green bell pepper, seeded and chopped
½ teaspoon sea salt
1 small head cauliflower, grated
1 cup corn kernels
½ cup prepared salsa
1 cup shredded pepper Jack cheese

1. In a large nonstick skillet over medium-high heat, heat the olive oil until it shimmers.
2. Add the turkey. Cook, crumbling with a spoon, until browned, about 5 minutes.
3. Add the onion, bell pepper, and salt. Cook, stirring occasionally, until the vegetables soften, 4 to 5 minutes.
4. Add the cauliflower, corn, and salsa. Cook, stirring, until the cauliflower rice softens, about 3 minutes more.
5. Sprinkle with the cheese. Reduce heat to low, cover, and allow the cheese to melt, 2 or 3 minutes.

Per Serving
calories: 448 | fat: 30g | protein: 30g | carbs: 18g | sugars: 5g | fiber: 4g | sodium: 649mg

Turkey Meatloaf Meatballs

Prep time: 10 minutes | Cook time: 20 minutes | Serves 4

¼ cup tomato paste
1 tablespoon honey
1 tablespoon Worcestershire sauce
½ cup milk
½ cup whole-wheat bread crumbs
1 pound (454 g)
ground turkey
1 onion, grated
1 tablespoon Dijon mustard
1 teaspoon dried thyme
½ teaspoon sea salt

1. Preheat the oven to 375ºF (190ºC). Line a rimmed baking sheet with parchment paper.
2. In a small saucepan on medium-low heat, whisk together the tomato paste, honey, and Worcestershire sauce. Bring to a simmer and then remove from the heat.
3. In a large bowl, combine the milk and bread crumbs. Let rest for 5 minutes.
4. Add the ground turkey, onion, mustard, thyme, and salt. Using your hands, mix well without overmixing.
5. Form into 1-inch meatballs and place on the prepared baking sheet. Brush the tops with the tomato paste mixture.
6. Bake until the meatballs reach 165ºF (74ºC) internally, about 15 minutes.

Per Serving
calories: 285 | fat: 11g | protein: 24g | carbs: 22g | sugars: 9g | fiber: 2g | sodium: 465mg

Turkey and Quinoa Caprese Casserole

Prep time: 10 minutes | Cook time: 35 minutes | Serves 8

⅔ cup quinoa
1⅓ cups water
Nonstick cooking spray
2 teaspoons extra-virgin olive oil
1 pound (454 g) lean ground turkey
¼ cup chopped red onion
½ teaspoon salt
1 (15-ounce / 425-g) can fire-roasted tomatoes, drained
4 cups spinach leaves, finely sliced
3 garlic cloves, minced
¼ cup sliced fresh basil
¼ cup chicken or vegetable broth
2 large ripe tomatoes, sliced
4 ounces (113 g) Mozzarella cheese, thinly sliced

1. In a small pot, combine the quinoa and water. Bring to a boil, reduce the heat, cover, and simmer for 10 minutes. Turn off the heat, and let the quinoa sit for 5 minutes to absorb any remaining water.
2. Preheat the oven to 400ºF (205ºC). Spray a baking dish with nonstick cooking spray.
3. In a large skillet, heat the oil over medium heat. Add the turkey, onion, and salt. Cook until the turkey is cooked through and crumbled.
4. Add the tomatoes, spinach, garlic, and basil. Stir in the broth and cooked quinoa. Transfer the mixture to the prepared baking dish. Arrange the tomato and cheese slices on top.
5. Bake for 15 minutes until the cheese is melted and the tomatoes are softened. Serve.

Per Serving
calories: 218 | fat: 9g | protein: 18g | carbs: 17g | sugars: 3g | fiber: 3g | sodium: 340mg

Chicken with Lemon Caper Pan Sauce

Prep time: 10 minutes | Cook time: 15 minutes | Serves 4

3 tablespoons extra-virgin olive oil
4 chicken breast halves or thighs, pounded slightly to even thickness
½ teaspoon sea salt
⅛ teaspoon freshly ground black pepper
¼ cup freshly squeezed lemon juice
¼ cup dry white wine
2 tablespoons capers, rinsed
2 tablespoons salted butter, very cold, cut into pieces

1. In a large skillet over medium-high heat, heat the olive oil until it shimmers.
2. Season the chicken with the salt and pepper. Add it to the hot oil and cook until opaque with an internal temperature of 165ºF (74ºC), about 5 minutes per side. Transfer the chicken to a plate and tent loosely with foil to keep warm. Keep the pan on the heat.
3. Add the lemon juice and wine to the pan, using the side of a spoon to scrape any browned bits from the bottom of the pan. Add the capers. Simmer until the liquid is reduced by half, about 3 minutes. Reduce the heat to low.
4. Whisk in the butter, one piece at a time, until incorporated.
5. Return the chicken to the pan, turning once to coat with the sauce. Serve with additional sauce spooned over the top.

Per Serving
calories: 281 | fat: 17g | protein: 26g | carbs: 2g | sugars: 0g | fiber: 0g | sodium: 386mg

Baked Chicken Tenders

Prep time: 10 minutes | Cook time: 15 minutes | Serves 4

1 cup whole-wheat bread crumbs
1 tablespoon dried thyme
1 teaspoon garlic powder
1 teaspoon paprika
½ teaspoon sea salt
3 large eggs, beaten
1 tablespoon Dijon mustard
1 pound (454 g) chicken, cut into ½-inch-thick pieces and pounded to even thickness

1. Preheat the oven to 375ºF (190ºC). Line a rimmed baking sheet with parchment paper.
2. In a medium bowl, whisk together the bread crumbs, thyme, garlic powder, paprika, and salt.
3. In another bowl, whisk together the eggs and mustard.
4. Dip each piece of chicken in the egg mixture and then in the bread crumb mixture. Place on the prepared baking sheet.
5. Bake until the chicken reaches an internal temperature of 165ºF (74ºC) and the bread crumbs are golden, about 15 minutes.

Per Serving
calories: 276 | fat: 6g | protein: 34g | carbs: 17g | sugars: 0g | fiber: 3g | sodium: 487mg

Coconut Chicken Curry

Prep time: 15 minutes | Cook time: 35 minutes | Serves 4

2 teaspoons extra-virgin olive oil
3 (5-ounce / 142-g) boneless, skinless chicken breasts, cut into 1-inch chunks
1 tablespoon grated fresh ginger
1 tablespoon minced garlic
2 tablespoons curry powder
2 cups low-sodium chicken broth
1 cup canned coconut milk
1 carrot, peeled and diced
1 sweet potato, diced
2 tablespoons chopped fresh cilantro

1. Place a large saucepan over medium-high heat and add the oil.
2. Sauté the chicken until lightly browned and almost cooked through, about 10 minutes.
3. Add the ginger, garlic, and curry powder, and sauté until fragrant, about 3 minutes.
4. Stir in the chicken broth, coconut milk, carrot, and sweet potato and bring the mixture to a boil.
5. Reduce the heat to low and simmer, stirring occasionally, until the vegetables and chicken are tender, about 20 minutes.
6. Stir in the cilantro and serve.

Per Serving
calories: 327 | fat: 17g | protein: 29g | carbs: 15g | sugars: 4g | fiber: 1g | sodium: 276mg

Ginger Citrus Chicken Thighs

Prep time: 15 minutes | Cook time: 30 minutes | Serves 4

4 chicken thighs, bone-in, skinless
1 tablespoon grated fresh ginger
Sea salt, to taste
1 tablespoon extra-virgin olive oil
Juice and zest of ½ lemon
Juice and zest of ½

orange
2 tablespoons honey
1 tablespoon reduced-sodium soy sauce
Pinch red pepper flakes
1 tablespoon chopped fresh cilantro

1. Rub the chicken thighs with the ginger and season lightly with salt.
2. Place a large skillet over medium-high heat and add the oil.
3. Brown the chicken thighs, turning once, for about 10 minutes.
4. While the chicken is browning, stir together the lemon juice and zest, orange juice and zest, honey, soy sauce, and red pepper flakes in a small bowl.
5. Add the citrus mixture to the skillet, cover, and reduce the heat to low.
6. Braise until the chicken is cooked through, about 20 minutes, adding a couple of tablespoons of water if the pan is too dry.
7. Serve garnished with the cilantro.

Per Serving
calories: 114 | fat: 5g | protein: 9g | carbs: 9g | sugars: 10g | fiber: 0g | sodium: 287mg

Asian Chicken Stir-Fry

Prep time: 10 minutes | Cook time: 10 minutes | Serves 4

3 tablespoons extra-virgin olive oil
1 pound (454 g) chicken breasts or thighs, cut into ¾-inch pieces
2 cups edamame or pea pods
3 garlic cloves, chopped
1 tablespoon peeled and grated fresh

ginger
2 tablespoons reduced-sodium soy sauce
Juice of 2 limes
1 teaspoon sesame oil
2 teaspoons toasted sesame seeds
1 tablespoon chopped fresh cilantro

1. In a large skillet over medium-high heat, heat the olive oil until it shimmers. Add the chicken to the oil and cook, stirring occasionally, until opaque, about 5 minutes. Add the edamame and cook, stirring occasionally, until crisp-tender, 3 to 5 minutes. Add the garlic and ginger and cook, stirring constantly, for 30 seconds.
2. In a small bowl, whisk together the soy sauce, lime juice, and sesame oil. Add the sauce mixture to the pan. Bring to a simmer, stirring, and cook for 2 minutes.
3. Remove from heat and garnish with the sesame seeds and cilantro.

Per Serving
calories: 331 | fat: 17g | protein: 31g | carbs: 11g | sugars: 0g | fiber: 5g | sodium: 342mg

Turkey Meatloaf Muffins

Prep time: 10 minutes | Cook time: 35 minutes | Serves 12

Nonstick cooking spray
½ cup old-fashioned oats
1 pound (454 g) lean ground turkey
½ cup finely chopped onion
1 red bell pepper,

seeded and finely chopped
2 eggs
3 garlic cloves, minced
1 teaspoon salt
½ teaspoon freshly ground black pepper

1. Preheat the oven to 375ºF (190ºC). Lightly spray a 12-cup muffin tin with nonstick cooking spray.
2. In a blender, process the oats until they become flour.
3. In a large mixing bowl, combine the oat flour, turkey, onion, bell pepper, eggs, and garlic. Mix well and season with the salt and pepper.
4. Using an ice cream scoop, transfer a ¼-cup portion of the meat mixture to each muffin cup.
5. Bake for 30 to 35 minutes until the muffins are cooked through.
6. Slide a knife along the outside of each cup to loosen the muffins and remove. Serve warm.

Per Serving
calories: 89 | fat: 4g | protein: 9g | carbs: 4g | sugars: 4g | fiber: 1g | sodium: 203mg

Orange Chicken

Prep time: 10 minutes | Cook time: 10 minutes | Serves 4

3 tablespoons extra-virgin olive oil
1 pound (454 g) chicken breasts or thighs, cut into ¾-inch pieces
1 teaspoon peeled and grated fresh ginger
2 garlic cloves, minced
1 tablespoon honey
Juice and zest of 1 orange
1 teaspoon cornstarch
½ teaspoon sriracha (or to taste)
Sesame seeds (optional, for garnish)
Thinly sliced scallion (optional, for garnish)

1. In a large skillet over medium-high heat, heat the olive oil until it shimmers. Add the chicken to the oil and cook, stirring occasionally, until opaque, about 5 minutes. Add the ginger and garlic and cook, stirring constantly, for 30 seconds.
2. In a small bowl, whisk together the honey, orange juice and zest, cornstarch, and sriracha. Add the sauce mixture to the chicken and cook, stirring, until the sauce thickens, about 2 minutes.
3. Serve garnished with sesame seeds and sliced scallions, if desired.

Per Serving
calories: 245 | fat: 12g | protein: 26g | carbs: 9g | sugars: 4g | fiber: 0g | sodium: 75mg

Chicken and Roasted Vegetable Wraps

Prep time: 10 minutes | Cook time: 20 minutes | Serves 4

½ small eggplant, cut into ¼-inch-thick slices
1 red bell pepper, seeded and cut into 1-inch-wide strips
1 medium zucchini, cut lengthwise into strips
½ small red onion, sliced
1 tablespoon extra-virgin olive oil
Sea salt and freshly ground black pepper, to taste
2 (8-ounce / 227-g) cooked chicken breasts, sliced
4 whole-wheat tortilla wraps

1. Preheat the oven to 400ºF (205ºC).
2. Line a baking sheet with aluminum foil and set it aside.
3. In a large bowl, toss the eggplant, bell pepper, zucchini, and red onion with the olive oil.
4. Transfer the vegetables to the baking sheet and lightly season with salt and pepper.
5. Roast the vegetables until soft and slightly charred, about 20 minutes.
6. Divide the vegetables and chicken into four portions.
7. Wrap 1 tortilla around each portion of chicken and grilled vegetables, and serve.

Per Serving
calories: 483 | fat: 25g | protein: 20g | carbs: 45g | sugars: 4g | fiber: 3g | sodium: 730mg

One-Pot Roast Chicken Dinner

Prep time: 10 minutes | Cook time: 40 minutes | Serves 6

½ head cabbage, cut into 2-inch chunks
1 sweet onion, peeled and cut into eighths
1 sweet potato, peeled and cut into 1-inch chunks
4 garlic cloves, peeled and lightly crushed
2 tablespoons extra-virgin olive oil, divided
2 teaspoons minced fresh thyme
Sea salt and freshly ground black pepper, to taste
2½ pounds (1.1 kg) bone-in chicken thighs and drumsticks

1. Preheat the oven to 450ºF (235ºC).
2. Lightly grease a large roasting pan and arrange the cabbage, onion, sweet potato, and garlic in the bottom. Drizzle with 1 tablespoon of oil, sprinkle with the thyme, and season the vegetables lightly with salt and pepper.
3. Season the chicken with salt and pepper.
4. Place a large skillet over medium-high heat and brown the chicken on both sides in the remaining 1 tablespoon of oil, about 10 minutes in total.
5. Place the browned chicken on top of the vegetables in the roasting pan. Roast until the chicken is cooked through, about 30 minutes.

Per Serving
calories: 540 | fat: 34g | protein: 43g | carbs: 14g | sugars: 5g | fiber: 4g | sodium: 242mg

Shredded Buffalo Chicken

Prep time: 10 minutes | Cook time: 27 minutes | Serves 8

2 tablespoons avocado oil
½ cup finely chopped onion
1 celery stalk, finely chopped
1 large carrot, chopped
⅓ cup mild hot sauce

½ tablespoon apple cider vinegar
¼ teaspoon garlic powder
2 bone-in, skin-on chicken breasts (about 2 pounds / 907 g)

1. Set the electric pressure cooker to the Sauté setting. When the pot is hot, pour in the avocado oil.
2. Sauté the onion, celery, and carrot for 3 to 5 minutes or until the onion begins to soften. Hit Cancel.
3. Stir in the hot sauce, vinegar, and garlic powder. Place the chicken breasts in the sauce, meat-side down.
4. Close and lock the lid of the pressure cooker. Set the valve to sealing.
5. Cook on high pressure for 20 minutes.
6. When cooking is complete, hit Cancel and quick release the pressure. Once the pin drops, unlock and remove the lid.
7. Using tongs, transfer the chicken breasts to a cutting board. When the chicken is cool enough to handle, remove the skin, shred the chicken and return it to the pot. Let the chicken soak in the sauce for at least 5 minutes.
8. Serve immediately.

Per Serving (½ cup)
calories: 139 | fat: 9g | protein: 12g | carbs: 2g | sugars: 1g | fiber: 1g | sodium: 295mg

Juicy Turkey Burgers

Prep time: 10 minutes | Cook time: 20 minutes | Serves 4

1½ pounds (680 g) lean ground turkey
½ cup bread crumbs
½ sweet onion, chopped
1 carrot, peeled, grated
1 teaspoon minced

garlic
1 teaspoon chopped fresh thyme
Sea salt and freshly ground black pepper, to taste
Nonstick cooking spray

1. In a large bowl, mix together the turkey, bread crumbs, onion, carrot, garlic, and thyme until very well mixed.
2. Season the mixture lightly with salt and pepper.
3. Shape the turkey mixture into 4 equal patties.
4. Place a large skillet over medium-high heat and coat it lightly with cooking spray.
5. Cook the turkey patties until golden and completely cooked through, about 10 minutes per side.
6. Serve the burgers plain or with your favorite toppings on a whole-wheat bun.

Per Serving
calories: 317 | fat: 15g | protein: 32g | carbs: 12g | sugars: 2g | fiber: 1g | sodium: 270mg

Smothered Burritos

Prep time: 5 minutes | Cook time: 20 minutes | Serves 4

Avocado oil cooking spray
½ small yellow onion, chopped
1 red bell pepper, chopped
1 pound (454 g) 93% lean ground turkey
1 teaspoon dried oregano

½ teaspoon smoked paprika
½ teaspoon garlic powder
8 medium yellow corn tortillas
1¼ cups jarred salsa or pico de gallo
¾ cup shredded Cheddar cheese

1. Heat a medium skillet over medium-low heat. When hot, coat the cooking surface with cooking spray, and place the onion, pepper, and ground turkey in the skillet.
2. Season the turkey with the oregano, smoked paprika, and garlic powder, and stir. Cook for 7 minutes.
3. Spoon ¼ cup of turkey into each tortilla. Wrap each tortilla into a burrito, then place the burritos seam-side down in a casserole dish. Pour the salsa over the burritos.
4. If your broiler is in the top of your oven, set the rack in the middle position. Set the broiler to high.
5. Top the burritos with the cheese, and broil for 4 minutes, or until the cheese is melted.

Per Serving
calories: 384 | fat: 16g | protein: 31g | carbs: 28g | sugars: 5g | fiber: 4g | sodium: 377mg

Firecracker Chicken Meatballs

Prep time: 15 minutes | Cook time: 21 minutes | Serves 6

Sauce:

½ cup hot sauce
2 tablespoons honey
2 tablespoons low-

sodium soy sauce or
tamari

Meatballs:

1 pound (454 g) ground chicken or turkey
1 cup Panko breadcrumbs (whole wheat, if possible)
1 large egg, slightly beaten

1½ teaspoons garlic pepper
1 teaspoon onion powder
¼ teaspoon kosher salt
2 tablespoons avocado oil, divided

Make the Sauce

1. In a 1-cup measuring cup, whisk together the hot sauce, honey, and soy sauce.

Make the Meatballs

1. In a large bowl, combine the chicken, Panko, egg, garlic pepper, onion powder, and salt. Mix gently with your hands until just combined. (Do not overmix or your meatballs will be tough.)
2. Pinch off about a tablespoon of the meat mixture and roll it into a ball. (A 1½-inch cookie scoop makes the job easy.) Repeat with the remaining meat. You should end up with about 30 (1½-inch) meatballs.
3. Set the electric pressure cooker to the Sauté/More setting. When the pot is hot, pour in 1 tablespoon of avocado oil.
4. Add half of the meatballs around the edge of the pot and brown them for 3 to 5 minutes. (The oil tends to pool towards the outside of the pot, so the meatballs will get browner if you put them there. Leaving space in the middle of the pot will also make it easier to turn the meatballs.) Flip the meatballs over and brown the other side for 3 to 5 minutes. Transfer to a paper towel-lined plate and repeat with the remaining 1 tablespoon of avocado oil and meatballs. Hit Cancel.
5. Return the meatballs to the pot and pour in the sauce mixture. Stir to coat all sides of the meatballs with sauce, then arrange them in a single layer.
6. Close and lock the lid of the pressure cooker. Set the valve to sealing.
7. Cook on high pressure for 6 minutes.
8. When the cooking is complete, hit Cancel. Allow the pressure to release naturally for 10 minutes, then quick release any remaining pressure.
9. Once the pin drops, unlock and remove the lid. Stir to evenly distribute the sauce.
10. Serve with toothpicks as an appetizer or as a main dish.

Per Serving (5 meatballs)
calories: 244 | fat: 12g | protein: 18g | carbs: 17g | sugars: 7g | fiber: 2g | sodium: 989mg

Herbed Whole Turkey Breast

Prep time: 10 minutes | Cook time: 30 minutes | Serves 12

3 tablespoons extra-virgin olive oil
1½ tablespoons herbes de Provence or poultry seasoning
2 teaspoons minced garlic
1 teaspoon lemon zest (from 1 small

lemon)
1 tablespoon kosher salt
1½ teaspoons freshly ground black pepper
1 (6-pound / 2.7-kg) bone-in, skin-on whole turkey breast, rinsed and patted dry

1. In a small bowl, whisk together the olive oil, herbes de Provence, garlic, lemon zest, salt, and pepper.
2. Rub the outside of the turkey and under the skin with the olive oil mixture.
3. Pour 1 cup of water into the electric pressure cooker and insert a wire rack or trivet.
4. Place the turkey on the rack, skin-side up.
5. Close and lock the lid of the pressure cooker. Set the valve to sealing.
6. Cook on high pressure for 30 minutes.
7. When the cooking is complete, hit Cancel. Allow the pressure to release naturally for 20 minutes, then quick release any remaining pressure.
8. Once the pin drops, unlock and remove the lid.
9. Carefully transfer the turkey to a cutting board. Remove the skin, slice, and serve.

Per Serving
calories: 146 | fat: 9g | protein: 16g | carbs: 0g | sugars: 0g | fiber: 0g | sodium: 413mg

Chicken Cacciatore

Prep time: 10 minutes | Cook time: 45 minutes | Serves 6

3 teaspoons extra-virgin olive oil, divided
6 chicken legs
8 ounces (227 g) brown mushrooms
1 large onion, sliced
1 red bell pepper, seeded and cut into strips
3 garlic cloves, minced
½ cup dry red wine
1 (28-ounce / 794-g) can whole tomatoes, drained
1 thyme sprig
1 rosemary sprig
½ teaspoon salt
¼ teaspoon freshly ground black pepper
¼ cup water

1. Preheat the oven to 350ºF (180ºC).
2. In a Dutch oven (or any oven-safe covered pot), heat 2 teaspoons of oil over medium-high heat. Sear the chicken on all sides until browned. Remove and set aside.
3. Heat the remaining 1 teaspoon of oil in the Dutch oven and sauté the mushrooms for 3 to 5 minutes until they brown and begin to release their water. Add the onion, bell pepper, and garlic, and mix together with the mushrooms. Cook an additional 3 to 5 minutes until the onion begins to soften.
4. Add the red wine and deglaze the pot. Bring to a simmer. Add the tomatoes, breaking them into pieces with a spoon. Add the thyme, rosemary, salt, and pepper to the pot and mix well.
5. Add the water, then nestle the cooked chicken, along with any juices that have accumulated, in the vegetables.
6. Transfer the pot to the oven. Cook for 30 minutes until the chicken is cooked through and its juices run clear. Remove the thyme and rosemary sprigs and serve.

Per Serving
calories: 257 | fat: 11g | protein: 28g | carbs: 11g | sugars: 6g | fiber: 2g | sodium: 398mg

Chicken Satay with Peanut Sauce

Prep time: 20 minutes | Cook time: 10 minutes | Serves 8

Peanut Sauce:
1 cup natural peanut butter
2 tablespoons low-sodium tamari or gluten-free soy sauce
1 teaspoon red chili paste
1 tablespoon honey
Juice of 2 limes
½ cup hot water

Chicken:
2 pounds (907 g) boneless, skinless chicken thighs, trimmed of fat and cut into 1-inch pieces
½ cup plain nonfat Greek yogurt
2 garlic cloves, minced
1 teaspoon minced fresh ginger
½ onion, coarsely chopped
1½ teaspoons ground coriander
2 teaspoons ground cumin
½ teaspoon salt
1 teaspoon extra-virgin olive oil
Lettuce leaves, for serving

Make the Peanut Sauce
1. In a medium mixing bowl, combine the peanut butter, tamari, chili paste, honey, lime juice, and hot water. Mix until smooth. Set aside.

Make the Chicken
1. In a large mixing bowl, combine the chicken, yogurt, garlic, ginger, onion, coriander, cumin, and salt, and mix well.
2. Cover and marinate in the refrigerator for at least 2 hours.
3. Thread the chicken pieces onto bamboo skewers.
4. In a grill pan or large skillet, heat the oil. Cook the skewers for 3 to 5 minutes on each side until the pieces are cooked through.
5. Remove the chicken from the skewers and place a few pieces on each lettuce leaf. Drizzle with the peanut sauce and serve.

Per Serving
calories: 386 | fat: 26g | protein: 30g | carbs: 14g | sugars: 6g | fiber: 2g | sodium: 442mg

Brown Mushroom Stuffed Turkey Breast

Prep time: 10 minutes | Cook time: 1 hour 5 minutes | Serves 8

2 tablespoons extra-virgin olive oil, divided
8 ounces (227 g) brown mushrooms, finely chopped
2 garlic cloves, minced
½ teaspoon salt, divided
¼ teaspoon freshly ground black pepper, divided
2 tablespoons chopped fresh sage
1 boneless, skinless turkey breast (about 3 pounds / 1.4 kg), butterflied

1. Preheat the oven to 375ºF (190ºC).
2. In a large skillet, heat 1 tablespoon of oil over medium heat. Add the mushrooms and cook for 4 to 5 minutes, stirring regularly, until most of the liquid has evaporated from the pan. Add the garlic, ¼ teaspoon of salt, and ⅛ teaspoon of pepper, and continue to cook for an additional minute. Add the sage to the pan, cook for 1 minute, and remove the pan from the heat.
3. On a clean work surface, lay the turkey breast flat. Use a kitchen mallet to pound the breast to an even 1-inch thickness throughout.
4. Spread the mushroom-sage mixture on the turkey breast, leaving a 1-inch border around the edges. Roll the breast tightly into a log.
5. Using kitchen twine, tie the breast two or three times around to hold it together. Rub the remaining 1 tablespoon of oil over the turkey breast. Season with the remaining ¼ teaspoon of salt and ⅛ teaspoon of pepper.
6. Transfer to a roasting pan and roast for 50 to 60 minutes, until the juices run clear, the meat is cooked through, and the internal temperature reaches 180ºF (82ºC).
7. Let rest for 5 minutes. Cut off the twine, slice, and serve.

Per Serving
calories: 232 | fat: 6g | protein: 41g | carbs: 2g | sugars: 0g | fiber: 0g | sodium: 320mg

Smoky Whole Chicken

Prep time: 20 minutes | Cook time: 21 minutes | Serves 6

2 tablespoons extra-virgin olive oil
1 tablespoon kosher salt
1½ teaspoons smoked paprika
1 teaspoon freshly ground black pepper
½ teaspoon herbes de Provence
¼ teaspoon cayenne pepper
1 (3½-pound / 1.6-kg) whole chicken, rinsed and patted dry,
giblets removed
1 large lemon, halved
6 garlic cloves, peeled and crushed with the flat side of a knife
1 large onion, cut into 8 wedges, divided
1 cup chicken bone broth, low-sodium store-bought chicken broth, or water
2 large carrots, each cut into 4 pieces
2 celery stalks, each cut into 4 pieces

1. In a small bowl, combine the olive oil, salt, paprika, pepper, herbes de Provence, and cayenne.
2. Place the chicken on a cutting board and rub the olive oil mixture under the skin and all over the outside. Stuff the cavity with the lemon halves, garlic cloves, and 3 to 4 wedges of onion.
3. Pour the broth into the electric pressure cooker. Add the remaining onion wedges, carrots, and celery. Insert a wire rack or trivet on top of the vegetables.
4. Place the chicken, breast-side up, on the rack.
5. Close and lock the lid of the pressure cooker. Set the valve to sealing.
6. Cook on high pressure for 21 minutes.
7. When the cooking is complete, hit Cancel and allow the pressure to release naturally for 15 minutes, then quick release any remaining pressure.
8. Once the pin drops, unlock and remove the lid.
9. Carefully remove the chicken to a clean cutting board. Remove the skin and cut the chicken into pieces or shred/chop the meat, and serve.

Per Serving
calories: 215 | fat: 9g | protein: 25g | carbs: 5g | sugars: 2g | fiber: 1g | sodium: 847mg

Braised Chicken with Grape-Apple Slaw

Prep time: 20 minutes | Cook time: 20 minutes | Serves 8

Chicken:

1 cup brown ale
1 teaspoon white wheat flour
2 bone-in, skin-on chicken breasts (about 2 pounds / 907 g)
Kosher salt and freshly ground black pepper, to taste
1 tablespoon coarse-grain mustard

Slaw:

¼ cup cider vinegar
2 tablespoons extra-virgin olive oil
1 tablespoon honey
1 tablespoon coarse-grain mustard
Kosher salt and freshly ground black pepper, to taste
¼ head purple or red cabbage, thinly sliced
2 cups seedless green grapes, halved
1 medium apple, cut into matchstick-size slices

Make the Chicken

1. In a 2-cup measuring cup or small bowl, whisk together the ale and flour. Pour into the electric pressure cooker.
2. Sprinkle the chicken breasts with salt and pepper. Place them in the electric pressure cooker, meat-side down.
3. Close and lock the lid of the pressure cooker. Set the valve to sealing.
4. Cook on high pressure for 20 minutes. While the chicken is cooking, make the slaw.
5. When the cooking is complete, hit Cancel. Allow the pressure to release naturally for 5 minutes, then quick release any remaining pressure.
6. Once the pin drops, unlock and remove the lid.
7. Using tongs, remove the chicken breasts to a cutting board. Hit Sauté/More and bring the liquid in the pot to a boil, scraping up any brown bits on the bottom of the pot. Cook, stirring occasionally, for about 5 minutes or until the sauce has reduced in volume by about a third. Hit Cancel and whisk in the mustard.
8. When the chicken is cool enough to handle, remove the skin, shred the meat, and return it to the pot. Let the chicken soak in the sauce for at least 5 minutes.
9. Serve the chicken topped with the slaw.

Make the Slaw

1. In a small jar with a screw-top lid, combine the vinegar, olive oil, honey, and mustard. Shake well, then season with salt and pepper, and shake again.
2. In a large bowl, toss together the cabbage, grapes, and apple. Add the dressing and mix well. Let the mixture sit at room temperature while the chicken cooks.

Per Serving (½ cup chicken, plus ½ cup slaw)
calories: 203 | fat: 9g | protein: 13g | carbs: 16g | sugars: 12g | fiber: 2g | sodium: 80mg

Chicken with Potatoes and Green Beans

Prep time: 5 minutes | Cook time: 30 minutes | Serves 4

⅓ cup low-sodium chicken broth
¼ cup extra-virgin olive oil
½ teaspoon salt
½ teaspoon freshly ground black pepper
¼ teaspoon garlic powder
¼ teaspoon dried thyme
1 teaspoon dried rosemary
4 (4-ounce / 113-g) boneless, skinless chicken breasts
4 small gold potatoes, cubed
1 pound (454 g) green beans

1. Preheat the oven to 400ºF (205ºC).
2. In a large bowl, whisk together the broth, oil, salt, pepper, garlic powder, thyme, and rosemary.
3. Add the chicken and potatoes to the marinade and coat well. Reserving the marinade, use a slotted spoon to remove the chicken and potatoes.
4. Arrange the chicken and potatoes on a baking sheet in a single layer and roast for 15 minutes.
5. Meanwhile, trim the green bean ends, if necessary, and put the beans in the reserved marinade.
6. Remove the baking sheet from the oven, flip the chicken breasts over, and add the green beans to the baking sheet. Pour the remaining marinade over the chicken.
7. Bake for 10 to 12 minutes until the chicken is cooked through, then broil for 2 minutes for a crisp, brown crust.

Per Serving
calories: 398 | fat: 15g | protein: 32g | carbs: 38g | sugars: 5g | fiber: 8g | sodium: 393mg

Hoisin Chicken Lettuce Wraps

Prep time: 10 minutes | Cook time: 20 minutes | Serves 4

Chicken:

2 teaspoons peanut oil

1/3 cup low-sodium gluten-free tamari or soy sauce

1 tablespoon honey

2 tablespoons rice vinegar

2 teaspoons Sriracha sauce

1 tablespoon minced garlic

2 teaspoons peeled and minced fresh ginger

1/3 cup chicken bone broth or water

2 scallions, both white and green parts, thinly sliced, divided

1 bone-in, skin-on chicken breast (about 1 pound / 454 g)

Lettuce Wraps:

Large lettuce leaves

1 cup broccoli slaw or shredded cabbage

1/4 cup chopped cashews, toasted

Make the Chicken

1. In the electric pressure cooker, whisk together the peanut oil, tamari, honey, rice vinegar, Sriracha, garlic, ginger, and broth. Stir in the white parts of the scallions.
2. Place the chicken breast in the sauce, meat-side down.
3. Close and lock the lid of the pressure cooker. Set the valve to sealing.
4. Cook on high pressure for 20 minutes.
5. When the cooking is complete, hit Cancel and quick release the pressure.
6. Once the pin drops, unlock and remove the lid.
7. Using tongs, transfer the chicken breast to a cutting board. When the chicken is cool enough to handle, remove the skin, shred the chicken, and return it to the pot. Let the chicken soak in the sauce for at least 5 minutes.

Make the Lettuce Wraps

1. Spoon some of the chicken and sauce into the lettuce leaves.
2. Sprinkle with the broccoli slaw, the green parts of the scallions, and the cashews.
3. Serve immediately.

Per Serving

calories: 233 | fat: 13g | protein: 14g | carbs: 18g | sugars: 10g | fiber: 2g | sodium: 1080mg

Sausage and Cauliflower "Grits"

Prep time: 7 minutes | Cook time: 20 minutes | Serves 4

1 pound (454 g) frozen (uncooked) Italian-style chicken or turkey sausages

1 pound (454 g) frozen riced cauliflower, broken up

1 tablespoon extra-virgin olive oil

Freshly ground black pepper, to taste

1/3 cup shredded Parmesan cheese

Chopped fresh parsley, for garnish

1. Pour 1/2 cup of water into the electric pressure cooker and add the sausages.
2. Close and lock the lid of the pressure cooker. Set the valve to sealing.
3. Cook on high pressure for 15 minutes.
4. When the cooking is complete, hit Cancel and quick release the pressure.
5. Once the pin drops, unlock and remove the lid.
6. Using tongs, transfer the sausages to a cutting board and slice into 1-inch rounds. Pour the liquid from the pot into a measuring cup. Pour 1/2 cup of the liquid back into the pot; discard the rest.
7. In the electric pressure cooker, combine the sliced sausage, cauliflower, olive oil, and pepper. Close and lock the lid of the pressure cooker. Set the valve to sealing.
8. Cook on high pressure for 5 minutes.
9. When the cooking is complete, hit Cancel and quick release the pressure.
10. Once the pin drops, unlock and remove the lid.
11. Stir in the Parmesan, garnish with parsley, and serve immediately.

Per Serving

calories: 263 | fat: 11g | protein: 30g | carbs: 111g | sugars: 4g | fiber: 3g | sodium: 660mg

Okra Stew with Chicken Andouille Sausage

Prep time: 10 minutes | Cook time: 30 minutes | Serves 4

3 tablespoons avocado oil, divided
½ large onion, halved and then cut into ¼-inch-thick slices
8 ounces (227 g) okra, cut into ½-inch-thick slices
¼ teaspoon kosher salt
¼ teaspoon freshly ground black pepper
3 garlic cloves, minced
1 teaspoon dried oregano

1 (28-ounce / 794-g) carton or can chopped tomatoes
2 links precooked chicken andouille sausage, cut into ¼-inch-thick slices (about 6 ounces / 170 g)
8 ounces (227 g) raw shrimp (26 to 35 count), peeled and deveined
Fresh parsley, chopped

1. Set the electric pressure cooker to the Sauté setting. When the pot is hot, pour in 1½ tablespoons avocado oil.
2. Add the onion and sauté for 3 to 5 minutes or until it begins to soften.
3. Add the remaining 1½ tablespoons olive oil and okra to the pot. Sprinkle with the salt and pepper. Sauté for 2 to 3 minutes or until the okra begins to brown a little bit. Hit Cancel.
4. Add the garlic, oregano, tomatoes and their juices, and 1 cup of water to the pot. Stir, then close and lock the lid of the pressure cooker. Set the valve to sealing.
5. Cook on high pressure for 20 minutes.
6. When the cooking is complete, hit Cancel and quick release the pressure.
7. Once the pin drops, unlock and remove the lid.
8. Hit Sauté and add the sausage and shrimp to the pot. Cook, uncovered, for about 5 minutes or until the shrimp is opaque and the sausage is hot.
9. Sprinkle with the parsley and serve.

Per Serving (1¼ cups)
calories: 252 | fat: 12g | protein: 16g | carbs: 24g | sugars: 10g | fiber: 6g | sodium: 732mg

Teriyaki Chicken and Broccoli

Prep time: 5 minutes | Cook time: 20 minutes | Serves 4

Sauce:
½ cup water
2 tablespoons low-sodium soy sauce
2 tablespoons honey
1 tablespoon rice vinegar

¼ teaspoon garlic powder
Pinch ground ginger
1 tablespoon cornstarch

Entrée:
1 tablespoon sesame oil
4 (4-ounce / 113-g) boneless, skinless chicken breasts, cut into bite-size cubes

1 (12-ounce / 340-g) bag frozen broccoli
1 (12-ounce / 340-g) bag frozen cauliflower rice

Make the Sauce
1. In a small saucepan, whisk together the water, soy sauce, honey, rice vinegar, garlic powder, and ginger. Add the cornstarch and whisk until it is fully incorporated.
2. Over medium heat, bring the teriyaki sauce to a boil. Let the sauce boil for 1 minute to thicken. Remove the sauce from the heat and set aside.

Make the Entrée
1. Heat a large skillet over medium-low heat. When hot, add the oil and the chicken. Cook for 5 to 7 minutes, until the chicken is cooked through, stirring as needed.
2. Steam the broccoli and cauliflower rice in the microwave according to the package instructions.
3. Divide the cauliflower rice into four equal portions. Put one-quarter of the broccoli and chicken over each portion and top with the teriyaki sauce.

Per Serving
calories: 247 | fat: 7g | protein: 29g | carbs: 20g | sugars: 12g | fiber: 5g | sodium: 418mg

Chicken Enchilada Spaghetti Squash

Prep time: 5 minutes | Cook time: 40 minutes | Serves 4

1 (3-pound / 1.4-kg) spaghetti squash, halved lengthwise and seeded
1½ teaspoons ground cumin, divided
Avocado oil cooking spray
4 (4-ounce / 113- g) boneless, skinless chicken breasts
1 large zucchini, diced
¾ cup canned red enchilada sauce
¾ cup shredded Cheddar or Mozzarella cheese

1. Preheat the oven to 400ºF (205ºC).
2. Season both halves of the squash with ½ teaspoon of cumin, and place them cut-side down on a baking sheet. Bake for 25 to 30 minutes.
3. Meanwhile, heat a large skillet over medium-low heat. When hot, spray the cooking surface with cooking spray and add the chicken breasts, zucchini, and 1 teaspoon of cumin. Cook the chicken for 4 to 5 minutes per side. Stir the zucchini when you flip the chicken.
4. Transfer the zucchini to a medium bowl and set aside. Remove the chicken from the skillet, and let it rest for 10 minutes or until it's cool enough to handle. Shred or dice the cooked chicken.
5. Place the chicken and zucchini in a large bowl, and add the enchilada sauce.
6. Remove the squash from the oven, flip it over, and comb through it with a fork to make thin strands.
7. Scoop the chicken mixture on top of the squash halves and top with the cheese. Return the squash to the oven and broil for 2 to 5 minutes, or until the cheese is bubbly.

Per Serving
calories: 331 | fat: 11g | protein: 35g | carbs: 27g | sugars: 2g | fiber: 4g | sodium: 491mg

Turkey Scaloppini

Prep time: 10 minutes | Cook time: 20 minutes | Serves 4

½ cup whole-wheat flour
½ teaspoon sea salt
¼ teaspoon freshly ground black pepper
3 tablespoons extra-virgin olive oil
12 ounces (340 g) turkey breast, cut into ½-inch-thick cutlets and pounded flat
1 garlic clove, minced
½ cup dry white wine
2 tablespoons chopped fresh rosemary
1 cup low-sodium chicken broth
2 tablespoons salted butter, very cold, cut into small pieces

1. Preheat the oven to 200ºF (93ºC). Line a baking sheet with parchment paper.
2. In a medium bowl, whisk together the flour, salt, and pepper.
3. In a large skillet over medium-high heat, heat the olive oil until it shimmers.
4. Working in batches with one or two pieces of turkey at a time (depending on how much room you have in the pan), dredge the turkey cutlets in the flour and pat off any excess. Cook in the hot oil until the turkey is cooked through, about 3 minutes per side. Add more oil if needed.
5. Place the cooked cutlets on the lined baking sheet and keep them warm in the oven while you cook the remaining turkey and make the pan sauce.
6. Once all the turkey is cooked and warming in the oven, add the garlic to the pan and cook, stirring constantly, for 30 seconds. Add the wine and use the side of a spoon to scrape any browned bits off the bottom of the pan. Simmer, stirring, for 1 minute. Add the rosemary and chicken broth. Simmer, stirring, until it thickens, 1 to 2 minutes more.
7. Whisk in the cold butter, one piece at a time, until incorporated. Return the turkey cutlets to the sauce and turn once to coat. Serve with any remaining sauce spooned over the top.

Per Serving
calories: 344 | fat: 20g | protein: 24g | carbs: 15g | sugars: 0g | fiber: 2g | sodium: 266mg

Spicy Chicken Cacciatore

Prep time: 20 minutes | Cook time: 1 hour | Serves 6

1 (2-pound / 907-g) chicken
¼ cup all-purpose flour
Sea salt and freshly ground black pepper, to taste
2 tablespoons extra-virgin olive oil
3 slices bacon, chopped
1 sweet onion, chopped
2 teaspoons minced garlic
4 ounces (113 g) button mushrooms, halved
1 (28-ounce / 794-g) can low-sodium stewed tomatoes
½ cup red wine
2 teaspoons chopped fresh oregano
Pinch red pepper flakes

1. Cut the chicken into pieces: 2 drumsticks, 2 thighs, 2 wings, and 4 breast pieces.
2. Dredge the chicken pieces in the flour and season each piece with salt and pepper.
3. Place a large skillet over medium-high heat and add the olive oil.
4. Brown the chicken pieces on all sides, about 20 minutes in total. Transfer the chicken to a plate.
5. Add the chopped bacon to the skillet and cook until crispy, about 5 minutes. With a slotted spoon, transfer the cooked bacon to the same plate as the chicken.
6. Pour off most of the oil from the skillet, leaving just a light coating. Sauté the onion, garlic, and mushrooms in the skillet until tender, about 4 minutes.
7. Stir in the tomatoes, wine, oregano, and red pepper flakes.
8. Bring the sauce to a boil. Return the chicken and bacon, plus any accumulated juices from the plate, to the skillet.
9. Reduce the heat to low and simmer until the chicken is tender, about 30 minutes.

Per Serving

calories: 230 | fat: 17g | protein: 8g | carbs: 14g | sugars: 5g | fiber: 2g | sodium: 420mg

Chicken with Creamy Thyme Sauce

Prep time: 15 minutes | Cook time: 30 minutes | Serves 4

4 (4-ounce / 113-g) boneless, skinless chicken breasts
Sea salt and freshly ground black pepper, to taste
1 tablespoon extra-virgin olive oil
½ sweet onion, chopped
1 cup low-sodium chicken broth
2 teaspoons chopped fresh thyme
¼ cup heavy (whipping) cream
1 tablespoon butter
1 scallion, white and green parts, chopped

1. Preheat the oven to 375ºF (190ºC).
2. Season the chicken breasts lightly with salt and pepper.
3. Place a large ovenproof skillet over medium-high heat and add the olive oil.
4. Brown the chicken, turning once, about 10 minutes in total. Transfer the chicken to a plate.
5. In the same skillet, sauté the onion until softened and translucent, about 3 minutes.
6. Add the chicken broth and thyme, and simmer until the liquid has reduced by half, about 6 minutes.
7. Stir in the cream and butter, and return the chicken and any accumulated juices from the plate to the skillet.
8. Transfer the skillet to the oven. Bake until cooked through, about 10 minutes.
9. Serve topped with the chopped scallion.

Per Serving

calories: 287 | fat: 14g | protein: 34g | carbs: 4g | sugars: 1g | fiber: 1g | sodium: 184mg

Tantalizing Jerked Chicken

Prep time: 10 minutes | Cook time: 20 minutes | Serves 4

4 (5-ounce / 142-g) boneless, skinless chicken breasts
½ sweet onion, cut into chunks
2 habanero chile peppers, halved lengthwise, seeded
¼ cup freshly squeezed lime juice
2 tablespoons extra-virgin olive oil
1 tablespoon minced garlic
1 tablespoon ground
allspice
2 teaspoons chopped fresh thyme
1 teaspoon freshly ground black pepper
½ teaspoon ground nutmeg
¼ teaspoon ground cinnamon
2 cups fresh greens (such as arugula or spinach)
1 cup halved cherry tomatoes

1. Place two chicken breasts in each of two large resealable plastic bags. Set them aside.
2. Place the onion, habaneros, lime juice, olive oil, garlic, allspice, thyme, black pepper, nutmeg, and cinnamon in a food processor and pulse until very well blended.
3. Pour half the marinade into each bag with the chicken breasts. Squeeze out as much air as possible, seal the bags, and place them in the refrigerator for 4 hours.
4. Preheat a barbecue to medium-high heat.
5. Let the chicken sit at room temperature for 15 minutes and then grill, turning at least once, until cooked through, about 15 minutes total.
6. Let the chicken rest for about 5 minutes before serving. Divide the greens and tomatoes among four serving plates, and top with the chicken.

Per Serving
calories: 226 | fat: 9g | protein: 33g | carbs: 3g | sugars: 1g | fiber: 0g | sodium: 92mg

Turkey Stuffed Peppers

Prep time: 15 minutes | Cook time: 50 minutes | Serves 4

1 teaspoon extra-virgin olive oil, plus more for greasing the baking dish
1 pound (454 g) ground turkey breast
½ sweet onion, chopped
1 teaspoon minced garlic
1 tomato, diced
½ teaspoon chopped fresh basil
Sea salt and freshly ground black pepper, to taste
4 red bell peppers, tops cut off, seeded
2 ounces (57 g) low-sodium feta cheese

1. Preheat the oven to 350ºF (180ºC).
2. Lightly grease a 9-by-9-inch baking dish with olive oil and set it aside.
3. Place a large skillet over medium heat and add 1 teaspoon of olive oil.
4. Add the turkey to the skillet and cook until it is no longer pink, stirring occasionally to break up the meat and brown it evenly, about 6 minutes.
5. Add the onion and garlic and sauté until softened and translucent, about 3 minutes.
6. Stir in the tomato and basil. Season with salt and pepper.
7. Place the peppers cut-side up in the baking dish. Divide the filling into four equal portions and spoon it into the peppers.
8. Sprinkle the feta cheese on top of the filling.
9. Add ¼ cup of water to the dish and cover with aluminum foil.
10. Bake the peppers until they are soft and heated through, about 40 minutes.

Per Serving
calories: 280 | fat: 14g | protein: 24g | carbs: 14g | sugars: 9g | fiber: 4g | sodium: 271mg

Herb-Roasted Turkey and Vegetables

Prep time: 20 minutes | Cook time: 2 hours | Serves 6

2 teaspoons minced garlic
1 tablespoon chopped fresh parsley
1 teaspoon chopped fresh thyme
1 teaspoon chopped fresh rosemary
2 pounds (907 g) boneless, skinless whole turkey breast
3 teaspoons extra-virgin olive oil, divided

Sea salt and freshly ground black pepper, to taste
2 sweet potatoes, peeled and cut into 2-inch chunks
2 carrots, peeled and cut into 2-inch chunks
2 parsnips, peeled and cut into 2-inch chunks
1 sweet onion, peeled and cut into eighths

1. Preheat the oven to 350ºF (180ºC).
2. Line a large roasting pan with aluminum foil and set it aside.
3. In a small bowl, mix together the garlic, parsley, thyme, and rosemary.
4. Place the turkey breast in the roasting pan and rub it all over with 1 teaspoon of olive oil.
5. Rub the garlic-herb mixture all over the turkey and season lightly with salt and pepper.
6. Place the turkey in the oven and roast for 30 minutes.
7. While the turkey is roasting, toss the sweet potatoes, carrots, parsnips, onion, and the remaining 2 teaspoons of olive oil in a large bowl.
8. Remove the turkey from the oven and arrange the vegetables around it.
9. Roast until the turkey is cooked through (170ºF / 77ºC internal temperature) and the vegetables are lightly caramelized, about 1 ½ hours.

Per Serving
calories: 273 | fat: 3g | protein: 38g | carbs: 20g | sugars: 6g | fiber: 4g | sodium: 116mg

Italian Turkey Sausage Meatballs

Prep time: 15 minutes | Cook time: 20 to 30 minutes | Makes about 24 meatballs

1 pound (454 g) ground chicken
8 ounces (227 g) Italian turkey sausage (hot or sweet), casings removed
2/3 cup Italian-style breadcrumbs
2 teaspoons minced garlic
3 tablespoons

chopped fresh parsley
½ cup freshly grated Parmesan cheese
3 tablespoons nonfat milk
1 large egg, lightly beaten
1 teaspoon kosher salt
½ teaspoon freshly ground black pepper

1. Preheat the oven to 350ºF (180ºC).
2. In a large bowl, combine the chicken, sausage, breadcrumbs, garlic, parsley, Parmesan, milk, egg, salt, and pepper. Mix gently but thoroughly. (I like to use my hands.)
3. Line a sheet pan with parchment paper. Pinch off about 1 tablespoon of the meat mixture and roll it into a ball. A 1¼-inch cookie scoop makes the job easy. Place the meatball on the sheet pan and repeat with the remaining meat. You should end up with about 24 meatballs.
4. If you plan to eat the meatballs right away, bake them for 30 minutes or until they are lightly browned and cooked through. If you plan to freeze the meatballs, bake them for 20 minutes, then let them cool before freezing.

Per Serving (4 meatballs)
calories: 269 | fat: 13g | protein: 25g | carbs: 12g | sugars: 3g | fiber:1 g | sodium: 877mg

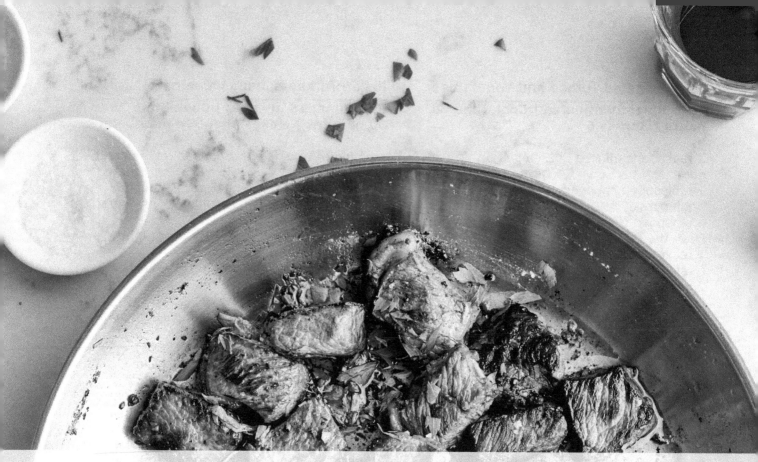
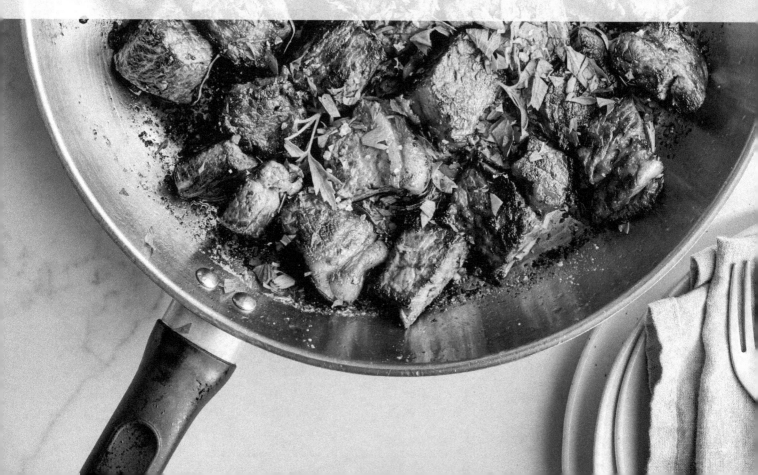

Chapter 7 Beef, Pork, and Lamb

Mustard Glazed Pork Chops

Prep time: 5 minutes | Cook time: 25 minutes | Serves 4

¼ cup Dijon mustard
1 tablespoon pure maple syrup
2 tablespoons rice vinegar
4 bone-in, thin-cut pork chops

1. Preheat the oven to 400ºF (205ºC).
2. In a small saucepan, combine the mustard, maple syrup, and rice vinegar. Stir to mix and bring to a simmer over medium heat. Cook for about 2 minutes until just slightly thickened.
3. In a baking dish, place the pork chops and spoon the sauce over them, flipping to coat.
4. Bake, uncovered, for 18 to 22 minutes until the juices run clear.

Per Serving
calories: 257 | fat: 7g | protein: 39g | carbs: 7g | sugars: 4g | fiber: 0g | sodium: 466mg

Parmesan-Crusted Pork Chops

Prep time: 10 minutes | Cook time: 25 minutes | Serves 4

Nonstick cooking spray
4 bone-in, thin-cut pork chops
2 tablespoons butter
½ cup grated Parmesan cheese
3 garlic cloves, minced
¼ teaspoon salt
¼ teaspoon dried thyme
Freshly ground black pepper, to taste

1. Preheat the oven to 400ºF (205ºC). Line a baking sheet with parchment paper and spray with nonstick cooking spray.
2. Arrange the pork chops on the prepared baking sheet so they do not overlap.
3. In a small bowl, combine the butter, cheese, garlic, salt, thyme, and pepper. Press 2 tablespoons of the cheese mixture onto the top of each pork chop.
4. Bake for 18 to 22 minutes until the pork is cooked through and its juices run clear. Set the broiler to high, then broil for 1 to 2 minutes to brown the tops.

Per Serving
calories: 332 | fat: 16g | protein: 44g | carbs: 1g | sugars: 0g | fiber: 0g | sodium: 440mg

Loaded Cottage Pie

Prep time: 15 minutes | Cook time: 1 hour | Serves 6 to 8

4 large russet potatoes, peeled and halved
3 tablespoons extra-virgin olive oil, divided
1 small onion, chopped
1 bunch collard greens, stemmed and thinly sliced
2 carrots, peeled and chopped
2 medium tomatoes, chopped
1 garlic clove, minced
1 pound (454 g) 90 percent lean ground beef
½ cup chicken broth
1 teaspoon Worcestershire sauce
1 teaspoon celery seeds
1 teaspoon smoked paprika
½ teaspoon dried chives
½ teaspoon ground mustard
½ teaspoon cayenne pepper

1. Preheat the oven to 400ºF (205ºC).
2. Bring a large pot of water to a boil.
3. Add the potatoes, and boil for 15 to 20 minutes, or until fork-tender.
4. Transfer the potatoes to a large bowl and mash with 1 tablespoon of olive oil.
5. In a large cast iron skillet, heat the remaining 2 tablespoons of olive oil.
6. Add the onion, collard greens, carrots, tomatoes, and garlic and sauté, stirring often, for 7 to 10 minutes, or until the vegetables are softened.
7. Add the beef, broth, Worcestershire sauce, celery seeds, and smoked paprika.
8. Spread the meat and vegetable mixture evenly onto the bottom of a casserole dish. Sprinkle the chives, ground mustard, and cayenne on top of the mixture. Spread the mashed potatoes evenly over the top.
9. Transfer the casserole dish to the oven, and bake for 30 minutes, or until the top is light golden brown.

Per Serving
calories: 440 | fat: 17g | protein: 27g | carbs: 48g | sugars: 6g | fiber: 9g | sodium: 107mg

Pulled Pork Sandwiches

Prep time: 5 minutes | Cook time: 15 minutes | Serves 4

Avocado oil cooking spray
8 ounces (227 g) store-bought pulled pork
½ cup chopped green bell pepper
2 slices provolone cheese
4 sandwich thins, 100% whole-wheat
2½ tablespoons apricot jelly

1. Heat the pulled pork according to the package instructions.
2. Heat a medium skillet over medium-low heat. When hot, coat the cooking surface with cooking spray.
3. Put the bell pepper in the skillet and cook for 5 minutes. Transfer to a small bowl and set aside.
4. Meanwhile, tear each slice of cheese into 2 strips, and halve the sandwich thins so you have a top and bottom.
5. Reduce the heat to low, and place the sandwich thins in the skillet cut-side down to toast, about 2 minutes.
6. Remove the sandwich thins from the skillet. Spread one-quarter of the jelly on the bottom half of each sandwich thin, then place one-quarter of the cheese, pulled pork, and pepper on top. Cover with the top half of the sandwich thin.

Per Serving
calories: 247 | fat: 8g | protein: 16g | carbs: 34g | sugars: 8g | fiber: 6g | sodium: 508mg

Roasted Pork Loin

Prep time: 5 minutes | Cook time: 40 minutes | Serves 4

1 pound (454 g) pork loin
1 tablespoon extra-virgin olive oil, divided
2 teaspoons honey
¼ teaspoon freshly ground black pepper
½ teaspoon dried
rosemary
2 small gold potatoes, chopped into 2-inch cubes
4 (6-inch) carrots, chopped into ½-inch rounds

1. Preheat the oven to 350ºF (180ºC).
2. Rub the pork loin with ½ tablespoon of oil and the honey. Season with the pepper and rosemary.
3. In a medium bowl, toss the potatoes and carrots in the remaining ½ tablespoon of oil.
4. Place the pork and the vegetables on a baking sheet in a single layer. Cook for 40 minutes.
5. Remove the baking sheet from the oven and let the pork rest for at least 10 minutes before slicing. Divide the pork and vegetables into four equal portions.

Per Serving
calories: 343 | fat: 10g | protein: 26g | carbs: 26g | sugars: 6g | fiber: 4g | sodium: 109mg

Open-Faced Philly Cheesesteak Sandwiches

Prep time: 5 minutes | Cook time: 25 minutes | Serves 4

Avocado oil cooking spray
1 cup chopped yellow onion
1 green bell pepper, chopped
12 ounces (340 g) 93% lean ground beef
Pinch salt
¾ teaspoon freshly ground black pepper
4 slices provolone or Swiss cheese
4 English muffins, 100% whole-wheat

1. Heat a large skillet over medium-low heat. When hot, coat the cooking surface with cooking spray, and arrange the onion and pepper in an even layer. Cook for 8 to 10 minutes, stirring every 3 to 4 minutes.
2. Push the vegetables to one side of the skillet and add the beef, breaking it into large chunks. Cook for 7 to 9 minutes, until a crisp crust forms on the bottom of the meat.
3. Season the beef with the salt and pepper, then flip the beef over and break it down into smaller chunks.
4. Stir the vegetables and the beef together, then top with the cheese and cook for 2 minutes.
5. Meanwhile, split each muffin in half, if necessary, then toast the muffins in a toaster.
6. Place one-eighth of the filling on each muffin half.

Per Serving
calories: 398 | fat: 16g | protein: 31g | carbs: 33g | sugars: 8g | fiber: 6g | sodium: 371mg

Lamb Burgers with Mushrooms and Cheese

Prep time: 15 minutes | Cook time: 15 minutes | Serves 4

8 ounces (227 g) grass-fed ground lamb
8 ounces (227 g) brown mushrooms, finely chopped
¼ teaspoon salt
¼ teaspoon freshly ground black pepper
¼ cup crumbled goat cheese
1 tablespoon minced fresh basil

1. In a large mixing bowl, combine the lamb, mushrooms, salt, and pepper, and mix well.
2. In a small bowl, mix the goat cheese and basil.
3. Form the lamb mixture into 4 patties, reserving about ½ cup of the mixture in the bowl. In each patty, make an indentation in the center and fill with 1 tablespoon of the goat cheese mixture. Use the reserved meat mixture to close the burgers. Press the meat firmly to hold together.
4. Heat the barbecue or a large skillet over medium-high heat. Add the burgers and cook for 5 to 7 minutes on each side, until cooked through. Serve.

Per Serving
calories: 173 | fat: 13g | protein: 11g | carbs: 3g | sugars: 1g | fiber: 0g | sodium: 154mg

Cherry-Glazed Lamb Chops

Prep time: 10 minutes | Cook time: 20 minutes | Serves 4

4 (4-ounce / 113-g) lamb chops
1½ teaspoons chopped fresh rosemary
¼ teaspoon salt
¼ teaspoon freshly ground black pepper
1 cup frozen cherries, thawed
¼ cup dry red wine
2 tablespoons orange juice
1 teaspoon extra-virgin olive oil

1. Season the lamb chops with the rosemary, salt, and pepper.
2. In a small saucepan over medium-low heat, combine the cherries, red wine, and orange juice, and simmer, stirring regularly, until the sauce thickens, 8 to 10 minutes.
3. Heat a large skillet over medium-high heat. When the pan is hot, add the olive oil to lightly coat the bottom.
4. Cook the lamb chops for 3 to 4 minutes on each side until well-browned yet medium rare.
5. Serve, topped with the cherry glaze.

Per Serving
calories: 356 | fat: 27g | protein: 20g | carbs: 6g | sugars: 4g | fiber: 1g | sodium: 199mg

Fresh Pot Pork Butt

Prep time: 10 minutes | Cook time: 45 minutes | Serves 8

2 tablespoons extra-virgin olive oil
¼ cup apple cider vinegar
1 tablespoon freshly ground black pepper
1 tablespoon dried oregano
1 small yellow onion, minced
2 scallions, white and green parts, minced
1 celery stalk, minced
Juice of 1 lime
2 pounds (907 g) boneless pork butt
4 garlic cloves, sliced
1 cup chicken broth

1. In a medium bowl, combine the oil, vinegar, pepper, oregano, onion, scallions, celery, and lime juice. Mix well until a paste is formed.
2. Score the pork with 1-inch-deep cuts in a diamond pattern on both sides. Push the garlic into the slits.
3. Massage the paste all over meat. Cover and refrigerate overnight or for at least 4 hours.
4. Select the Sauté setting on an electric pressure cooker. Cook the meat for 2 minutes on each side.
5. Add the broth, close and lock the lid, and set the pressure valve to sealing.
6. Change to the Manual setting, and cook for 20 minutes.
7. Once cooking is complete, allow the pressure to release naturally. Carefully remove the lid.
8. Remove the pork from the pressure cooker, and serve with Ranch Dressing.

Per Serving
calories: 287 | fat: 22g | protein: 20g | carbs: 1g | sugars: 1g | fiber: 1g | sodium: 88mg

Beef Curry

Prep time: 15 minutes | Cook time: 10 minutes | Serves 6

1 tablespoon extra-virgin olive oil
1 small onion, thinly sliced
2 teaspoons minced fresh ginger
3 garlic cloves, minced
2 teaspoons ground coriander
1 teaspoon ground cumin
1 jalapeño or serrano pepper, slit lengthwise
but not all the way through
¼ teaspoon ground turmeric
¼ teaspoon salt
1 pound (454 g) grass-fed sirloin tip steak, top round steak, or top sirloin steak, cut into bite-size pieces
2 tablespoons chopped fresh cilantro

1. In a large skillet, heat the oil over medium high.
2. Add the onion, and cook for 3 to 5 minutes until browned and softened. Add the ginger and garlic, stirring continuously until fragrant, about 30 seconds.
3. In a small bowl, mix the coriander, cumin, jalapeño, turmeric, and salt. Add the spice mixture to the skillet and stir continuously for 1 minute. Deglaze the skillet with about ¼ cup of water.
4. Add the beef and stir continuously for about 5 minutes until well-browned yet still medium rare. Remove the jalapeño. Serve topped with the cilantro.

Per Serving
calories: 140 | fat: 7g | protein: 18g | carbs: 3g | sugars: 1g | fiber: 1g | sodium: 141mg

Steak Fajita Bake

Prep time: 10 minutes | Cook time: 15 minutes | Serves 4

1 green bell pepper
1 yellow bell pepper
1 red bell pepper
1 small white onion
10 ounces (283 g) sirloin steak, trimmed of visible fat
2 tablespoons avocado oil
½ teaspoon ground cumin
¼ teaspoon chili powder
¼ teaspoon garlic powder
4 (6-inch) 100% whole-wheat tortillas

1. Preheat the oven to 400ºF (205ºC).
2. Cut the green bell pepper, yellow bell pepper, red bell pepper, onion, and steak into ½-inch-thick slices, and put them on a large baking sheet.
3. In a small bowl, combine the oil, cumin, chili powder, and garlic powder, then drizzle the mixture over the meat and vegetables to fully coat them.
4. Arrange the steak and vegetables in a single layer, and bake for 10 to 15 minutes, or until the steak is cooked through.
5. Divide the steak and vegetables equally between the tortillas.

Per Serving
calories: 349 | fat: 18g | protein: 19g | carbs: 28g | sugars: 5g | fiber: 5g | sodium: 197mg

Chipotle Chili Pork Chops

Prep time: 5 minutes | Cook time: 20 minutes | Serves 4

Juice and zest of 1 lime
1 tablespoon extra-virgin olive oil
1 tablespoon chipotle chili powder
2 teaspoons minced garlic
1 teaspoon ground cinnamon
Pinch sea salt
4 (5-ounce / 142-g) pork chops, about 1 inch thick
Lime wedges, for garnish

1. Combine the lime juice and zest, oil, chipotle chili powder, garlic, cinnamon, and salt in a resealable plastic bag. Add the pork chops. Remove as much air as possible and seal the bag.
2. Marinate the chops in the refrigerator for at least 4 hours, and up to 24 hours, turning them several times.
3. Preheat the oven to 400ºF (205ºC) and set a rack on a baking sheet. Let the chops rest at room temperature for 15 minutes, then arrange them on the rack and discard the remaining marinade.
4. Roast the chops until cooked through, turning once, about 10 minutes per side.
5. Serve with lime wedges.

Per Serving
calories: 204 | fat: 9g | protein: 30g | carbs: 1g | sugars: 1g | fiber: 0g | sodium: 317mg

Broccoli Beef Stir-Fry

Prep time: 10 minutes | Cook time: 15 minutes | Serves 4

2 tablespoons extra-virgin olive oil
1 pound (454 g) sirloin steak, cut into ¼-inch-thick strips
2 cups broccoli florets
1 garlic clove, minced
1 teaspoon peeled and grated fresh ginger
2 tablespoons reduced-sodium soy sauce
¼ cup beef broth
½ teaspoon Chinese hot mustard
Pinch red pepper flakes

1. In a large skillet over medium-high heat, heat the olive oil until it shimmers. Add the beef. Cook, stirring, until it browns, 3 to 5 minutes. With a slotted spoon, remove the beef from the oil and set it aside on a plate.
2. Add the broccoli to the oil. Cook, stirring, until it is crisp-tender, about 4 minutes.
3. Add the garlic and ginger and cook, stirring constantly, for 30 seconds.
4. Return the beef to the pan, along with any juices that have collected.
5. In a small bowl, whisk together the soy sauce, broth, mustard, and red pepper flakes.
6. Add the soy sauce mixture to the skillet and cook, stirring, until everything warms through, about 3 minutes.

Per Serving
calories: 227 | fat: 11g | protein: 27g | carbs: 5g | sugars: 0g | fiber: 1g | sodium: 375mg

Beef Burrito Bowl

Prep time: 5 minutes | Cook time: 15 minutes | Serves 4

1 pound (454 g) 93% lean ground beef
1 cup canned low-sodium black beans, drained and rinsed
¼ teaspoon ground cumin
¼ teaspoon chili powder
¼ teaspoon garlic powder
¼ teaspoon onion
powder
¼ teaspoon salt
1 head romaine or preferred lettuce, shredded
2 medium tomatoes, chopped
1 cup shredded Cheddar cheese or packaged cheese blend

1. Heat a large skillet over medium-low heat. Put the beef, beans, cumin, chili powder, garlic powder, onion powder, and salt into the skillet, and cook for 8 to 10 minutes, until cooked through. Stir occasionally.
2. Divide the lettuce evenly between four bowls. Add one-quarter of the beef mixture to each bowl and top with one-quarter of the tomatoes and cheese.

Per Serving
calories: 351 | fat: 18g | protein: 35g | carbs: 14g | sugars: 4g | fiber: 6g | sodium: 424mg

Bunless Sloppy Joes

Prep time: 15 minutes | Cook time: 40 minutes | Serves 6

6 small sweet potatoes
1 pound (454 g) lean ground beef
1 onion, finely chopped
1 carrot, finely chopped
¼ cup finely chopped mushrooms
¼ cup finely chopped red bell pepper
3 garlic cloves, minced
2 teaspoons Worcestershire sauce
1 tablespoon white wine vinegar
1 (15-ounce / 425-g) can low-sodium tomato sauce
2 tablespoons tomato paste

1. Preheat the oven to 400ºF (205ºC).
2. Place the sweet potatoes in a single layer in a baking dish. Bake for 25 to 40 minutes, depending on the size, until they are soft and cooked through.
3. While the sweet potatoes are baking, in a large skillet, cook the beef over medium heat until it's browned, breaking it apart into small pieces as you stir.
4. Add the onion, carrot, mushrooms, bell pepper, and garlic, and sauté briefly for 1 minute.
5. Stir in the Worcestershire sauce, vinegar, tomato sauce, and tomato paste. Bring to a simmer, reduce the heat, and cook for 5 minutes for the flavors to meld.
6. Scoop ½ cup of the meat mixture on top of each baked potato and serve.

Per Serving
calories: 372 | fat: 19g | protein: 16g | carbs: 34g | sugars: 13g | fiber: 6g | sodium: 161mg

Pork and Apple Skillet

Prep time: 10 minutes | Cook time: 20 minutes | Serves 4

1 pound (454 g) ground pork	thyme
1 red onion, thinly sliced	2 garlic cloves, minced
2 apples, peeled, cored, and thinly sliced	¼ cup apple cider vinegar
2 cups shredded cabbage	1 tablespoon Dijon mustard
1 teaspoon dried	½ teaspoon sea salt
	⅛ teaspoon freshly ground black pepper

1. In a large skillet over medium-high heat, cook the ground pork, crumbling it with a spoon, until browned, about 5 minutes. Use a slotted spoon to transfer the pork to a plate.
2. Add the onion, apples, cabbage, and thyme to the fat in the pan. Cook, stirring occasionally, until the vegetables are soft, about 5 minutes.
3. Add the garlic and cook, stirring constantly, for 5 minutes.
4. Return the pork to the pan.
5. In a small bowl, whisk together the vinegar, mustard, salt, and pepper. Add to the pan. Bring to a simmer. Cook, stirring, until the sauce thickens, about 2 minutes.

Per Serving

calories: 364 | fat: 24g | protein: 20g | carbs: 19g | sugars: g | fiber: 4g | sodium: 260mg

Beef and Pepper Fajita Bowls

Prep time: 10 minutes | Cook time: 15 minutes | Serves 4

4 tablespoons extra-virgin olive oil, divided	seeded and sliced
1 head cauliflower, riced	1 onion, thinly sliced
1 pound (454 g) sirloin steak, cut into ¼-inch-thick strips	2 garlic cloves, minced
1 red bell pepper,	Juice of 2 limes
	1 teaspoon chili powder

1. In a large skillet over medium-high heat, heat 2 tablespoons of olive oil until it shimmers. Add the cauliflower. Cook, stirring occasionally, until it softens, about 3 minutes. Set aside.

2. Wipe out the skillet with a paper towel. Add the remaining 2 tablespoons of oil to the skillet, and heat it on medium-high until it shimmers. Add the steak and cook, stirring occasionally, until it browns, about 3 minutes. Use a slotted spoon to remove the steak from the oil in the pan and set aside.
3. Add the bell pepper and onion to the pan. Cook, stirring occasionally, until they start to brown, about 5 minutes.
4. Add the garlic and cook, stirring constantly, for 30 seconds.
5. Return the beef along with any juices that have collected and the cauliflower to the pan. Add the lime juice and chili powder. Cook, stirring, until everything is warmed through, 2 to 3 minutes.

Per Serving

calories: 310 | fat: 18g | protein: 27g | carbs: 13g | sugars: 2g | fiber: 3g | sodium: 93mg

Slow Cooker Ropa Vieja

Prep time: 5 minutes | Cook time: 20 minutes | Serves 4

½ small yellow onion	½ teaspoon smoked paprika
1 red bell pepper	½ teaspoon garlic powder
1 (14-ounce / 397-g) can no-salt-added diced tomatoes	1 pound (454 g) chuck beef roast, trimmed of visible fat
1 teaspoon dried oregano	1 head cauliflower
½ teaspoon salt	

1. Cut the onion and bell pepper into ½-inch-thick slices.
2. Place the onion, bell pepper, diced tomatoes with their juices, oregano, salt, paprika, and garlic powder in a slow cooker, then add the beef.
3. Place the head of cauliflower on top of the beef, and cook on low for 8 hours.
4. When fully cooked, the cauliflower will fall apart when scooped.

Per Serving

calories: 356 | fat: 18g | protein: 35g | carbs: 15g | sugars: 7g | fiber: 5g | sodium: 420mg

Homestyle Herb Meatballs

Prep time: 10 minutes | Cook time: 15 minutes | Serves 4

½ pound (227 g) lean ground pork
½ pound (227 g) lean ground beef
1 sweet onion, finely chopped
¼ cup bread crumbs
2 tablespoons
chopped fresh basil
2 teaspoons minced garlic
1 egg
Pinch sea salt
Pinch freshly ground black pepper

1. Preheat the oven to 350°F (180°C).
2. Line a baking tray with parchment paper and set it aside.
3. In a large bowl, mix together the pork, beef, onion, bread crumbs, basil, garlic, egg, salt, and pepper until very well mixed.
4. Roll the meat mixture into 2-inch meatballs.
5. Transfer the meatballs to the baking sheet and bake until they are browned and cooked through, about 15 minutes.
6. Serve the meatballs with your favorite marinara sauce and some steamed green beans.

Per Serving
calories: 332 | fat: 19g | protein: 24g | carbs: 13g | sugars: 3g | fiber: 1g | sodium: 188mg

Lime-Parsley Lamb Cutlets

Prep time: 10 minutes | Cook time: 10 minutes | Serves 4

¼ cup extra-virgin olive oil
¼ cup freshly squeezed lime juice
2 tablespoons lime zest
2 tablespoons
chopped fresh parsley
Pinch sea salt
Pinch freshly ground black pepper
12 lamb cutlets (about 1½ pounds / 680 g total)

1. In a medium bowl, whisk together the oil, lime juice, zest, parsley, salt, and pepper.
2. Transfer the marinade to a resealable plastic bag.
3. Add the cutlets to the bag and remove as much air as possible before sealing.
4. Marinate the lamb in the refrigerator for about 4 hours, turning the bag several times.

5. Preheat the oven to broil.
6. Remove the chops from the bag and arrange them on an aluminum foil-lined baking sheet. Discard the marinade.
7. Broil the chops for 4 minutes per side for medium doneness.
8. Let the chops rest for 5 minutes before serving.

Per Serving
calories: 413 | fat: 29g | protein: 31g | carbs: 1g | sugars: 0g | fiber: 0g | sodium: 100mg

Mediterranean Steak Sandwiches

Prep time: 10 minutes | Cook time: 10 minutes | Serves 4

2 tablespoons extra-virgin olive oil
2 tablespoons balsamic vinegar
2 teaspoons minced garlic
2 teaspoons freshly squeezed lemon juice
2 teaspoons chopped fresh oregano
1 teaspoon chopped
fresh parsley
1 pound (454 g) flank steak, trimmed of fat
4 whole-wheat pitas
2 cups shredded lettuce
1 red onion, thinly sliced
1 tomato, chopped
1 ounce (28 g) low-sodium feta cheese

1. In a large bowl, whisk together the olive oil, balsamic vinegar, garlic, lemon juice, oregano, and parsley.
2. Add the steak to the bowl, turning to coat it completely.
3. Marinate the steak for 1 hour in the refrigerator, turning it over several times.
4. Preheat the broiler. Line a baking sheet with aluminum foil.
5. Take the steak out of the bowl and discard the marinade.
6. Place the steak on the baking sheet and broil until it is done to your liking, about 5 minutes per side for medium.
7. Let the steak rest for 10 minutes before slicing it thinly on a bias.
8. Stuff the pitas with the sliced steak, lettuce, onion, tomato, and feta.

Per Serving
calories: 344 | fat: 16g | protein: 28g | carbs: 22g | sugars: 3g | fiber: 3g | sodium: 296mg

Lamb Kofta Meatballs with Cucumber Salad

Prep time: 10 minutes | Cook time: 15 minutes | Serves 4

¼ cup red wine vinegar
Pinch red pepper flakes
1 teaspoon sea salt, divided
2 cucumbers, peeled and chopped
½ red onion, finely chopped

1 pound (454 g) ground lamb
2 teaspoons ground coriander
1 teaspoon ground cumin
3 garlic cloves, minced
1 tablespoon fresh mint, chopped

1. Preheat the oven to 375ºF (190ºC). Line a rimmed baking sheet with parchment paper.
2. In a medium bowl, whisk together the vinegar, red pepper flakes, and ½ teaspoon of salt. Add the cucumbers and onion and toss to combine. Set aside.
3. In a large bowl, mix the lamb, coriander, cumin, garlic, mint, and remaining ½ teaspoon of salt. Form the mixture into 1-inch meatballs and place them on the prepared baking sheet.
4. Bake until the lamb reaches 140ºF (60ºC) internally, about 15 minutes.
5. Serve with the salad on the side.

Per Serving
calories: 345 | fat: 27g | protein: 20g | carbs: 7g | sugars: 3g | fiber: 1g | sodium: 362mg

Traditional Beef Stroganoff

Prep time: 10 minutes | Cook time: 30 minutes | Serves 4

1 teaspoon extra-virgin olive oil
1 pound (454 g) top sirloin, cut into thin strips
1 cup sliced button mushrooms
½ sweet onion, finely chopped
1 teaspoon minced garlic
1 tablespoon whole-

wheat flour
½ cup low-sodium beef broth
¼ cup dry sherry
½ cup fat-free sour cream
1 tablespoon chopped fresh parsley
Sea salt and freshly ground black pepper, to taste

1. Place a large skillet over medium-high heat and add the oil.
2. Sauté the beef until browned, about 10 minutes, then remove the beef with a slotted spoon to a plate and set it aside.
3. Add the mushrooms, onion, and garlic to the skillet and sauté until lightly browned, about 5 minutes.
4. Whisk in the flour and then whisk in the beef broth and sherry.
5. Return the sirloin to the skillet and bring the mixture to a boil.
6. Reduce the heat to low and simmer until the beef is tender, about 10 minutes.
7. Stir in the sour cream and parsley. Season with salt and pepper.

Per Serving
calories: 257 | fat: 14g | protein: 26g | carbs: 6g | sugars: 1g | fiber: 1g | sodium: 141mg

Curried Pork and Vegetable Skewers

Prep time: 15 minutes | Cook time: 15 minutes | Serves 4

¼ cup plain nonfat Greek yogurt
2 tablespoons curry powder
1 teaspoon garlic powder
1 teaspoon ground turmeric
Zest and juice of 1 lime
¼ teaspoon salt
Pinch freshly ground black pepper

1 pound (454 g) boneless pork tenderloin, cut into bite-size pieces
1 red bell pepper, seeded and cut into 2-inch squares
1 green bell pepper, seeded and cut into 2-inch squares
1 red onion, quartered and split into segments

1. In a large bowl, mix the yogurt, curry powder, garlic powder, turmeric, lime zest, lime juice, salt, and pepper.
2. Add the pieces of pork tenderloin to the bowl, and stir to coat. Refrigerate for at least 1 hour or as long as 6 hours.
3. Preheat a grill or broiler to medium.
4. Thread the pork pieces, bell peppers, and onions onto skewers.
5. Grill or broil for 12 to 15 minutes, flipping every 3 or 4 minutes, until the pork is cooked through. Serve.

Per Serving
calories: 175 | fat: 3g | protein: 27g | carbs: 10g | sugars: 4g | fiber: 3g | sodium: 188mg

Smothered Sirloin

Prep time: 15 minutes | Cook time: 30 minutes | Serves 5

1 pound (454 g) beef round sirloin tip
1 teaspoon freshly ground black pepper
1 teaspoon celery seeds
2 tablespoons extra-virgin olive oil
1 medium yellow onion, chopped
¼ cup chickpea flour
2 cups chicken broth, divided
2 celery stalks, thinly sliced
1 medium red bell pepper, chopped
2 garlic cloves, minced
2 tablespoons whole-wheat flour
Generous pinch cayenne pepper
Chopped fresh chives, for garnish (optional)
Smoked paprika, for garnish (optional)

1. In a bowl, season the steak on both sides with the black pepper and celery seeds.
2. Select the Sauté setting on an electric pressure cooker, and combine the olive oil and onions. Cook for 3 to 5 minutes, stirring, or until the onions are browned but not burned.
3. Slowly add the chickpea flour, 1 tablespoon at a time, while stirring.
4. Add 1 cup of broth, ¼ cup at a time, as needed.
5. Stir in the celery, bell pepper, and garlic and cook for 3 to 5 minutes, or until softened.
6. Lay the beef on top of vegetables, and pour the remaining 1 cup of broth on top.
7. Close and lock the lid and set the pressure valve to sealing.
8. Change to the Manual setting, and cook for 20 minutes.
9. Once cooking is complete, quick-release the pressure. Carefully remove the lid.
10. Remove the steak and vegetables from the pressure cooker, reserving the leftover liquid for the gravy base.
11. To make the gravy, add the whole-wheat flour and cayenne to the liquid in the pressure cooker, mixing continuously until thickened.
12. To serve, spoon the gravy over the steak and garnish with the chives (if using) and paprika (if using).

Per Serving

calories: 253 | fat: 13g | protein: 22g | carbs: 10g | sugars: 3g | fiber: 2g | sodium: 86mg

Beef and Butternut Squash Stew

Prep time: 15 minutes | Cook time: 38 minutes | Serves 8

1½ tablespoons smoked paprika
2 teaspoons ground cinnamon
1½ teaspoons kosher salt
1 teaspoon ground ginger
1 teaspoon red pepper flakes
½ teaspoon freshly ground black pepper
2 pounds (907 g) beef shoulder roast, cut into 1-inch cubes
2 tablespoons avocado oil, divided
1 cup low-sodium beef or vegetable broth
1 medium red onion, cut into wedges
8 garlic cloves, minced
1 (28-ounce / 794-g) carton or can no-salt-added diced tomatoes
2 pounds (907 g) butternut squash, peeled and cut into 1-inch pieces
Chopped fresh cilantro or parsley, for serving

1. In a zip-top bag or medium bowl, combine the paprika, cinnamon, salt, ginger, red pepper, and black pepper. Add the beef and toss to coat.
2. Set the electric pressure cooker to the Sauté setting. When the pot is hot, pour in 1 tablespoon of avocado oil.
3. Add half of the beef to the pot and cook, stirring occasionally, for 3 to 5 minutes or until the beef is no longer pink. Transfer it to a plate, then add the remaining 1 tablespoon of avocado oil and brown the remaining beef. Transfer to the plate. Hit Cancel.
4. Stir in the broth and scrape up any brown bits from the bottom of the pot. Return the beef to the pot and add the onion, garlic, tomatoes and their juices, and squash. Stir well.
5. Close and lock lid of pressure cooker. Set the valve to sealing.
6. Cook on high pressure for 30 minutes.
7. When cooking is complete, hit Cancel. Allow the pressure to release naturally for 10 minutes, then quick release any remaining pressure.
8. Unlock and remove lid.
9. Spoon into serving bowls, sprinkle with cilantro or parsley, and serve.

Per Serving (1½ cups)

calories: 268 | fat: 10g | protein: 25g | carbs: 26g | sugars: 7g | fiber: 7g | sodium: 3887mg

Sunday Pot Roast

Prep time: 10 minutes | Cook time: 1 hour 45 minutes | Serves 10

1 (3- to 4-pound / 1.4- to 1.8-kg) beef rump roast
2 teaspoons kosher salt, divided
2 tablespoons avocado oil
1 large onion, coarsely chopped (about 1½ cups)
4 large carrots, each

cut into 4 pieces
1 tablespoon minced garlic
3 cups low-sodium beef broth
1 teaspoon freshly ground black pepper
1 tablespoon dried parsley
2 tablespoons all-purpose flour

1. Rub the roast all over with 1 teaspoon of the salt.
2. Set the electric pressure cooker to the Sauté setting. When the pot is hot, pour in the avocado oil.
3. Carefully place the roast in the pot and sear it for 6 to 9 minutes on each side. (You want a dark caramelized crust.) Hit Cancel.
4. Transfer the roast from the pot to a plate.
5. In order, put the onion, carrots, and garlic in the pot. Place the roast on top of the vegetables along with any juices that accumulated on the plate.
6. In a medium bowl, whisk together the broth, remaining 1 teaspoon of salt, pepper, and parsley. Pour the broth mixture over the roast.
7. Close and lock the lid of the pressure cooker. Set the valve to sealing.
8. Cook on high pressure for 1 hour and 30 minutes.
9. When the cooking is complete, hit Cancel and allow the pressure to release naturally.
10. Once the pin drops, unlock and remove the lid.
11. Using large slotted spoons, transfer the roast and vegetables to a serving platter while you make the gravy.
12. Using a large spoon or fat separator, remove the fat from the juices in the pot. Set the electric pressure cooker to the Sauté setting and bring the liquid to a boil.
13. In a small bowl, whisk together the flour and 4 tablespoons of water to make a slurry. Pour the slurry into the pot, whisking occasionally, until the gravy is the thickness you like. Season with salt and pepper, if necessary.
14. Serve the meat and carrots with the gravy.

Per Serving
calories: 245 | fat: 10g | protein: 33g | carbs: 6g | sugars: 2g | fiber: 1g | sodium: 397mg

Rosemary Lamb Chops

Prep time: 25 minutes | Cook time: 10 minutes | Serves 4

1½ pounds (680 g) lamb chops (4 small chops)
1 teaspoon kosher salt
Leaves from 1 (6-inch) rosemary sprig

2 tablespoons avocado oil
1 shallot, peeled and cut in quarters
1 tablespoon tomato paste
1 cup beef broth

1. Place the lamb chops on a cutting board. Press the salt and rosemary leaves into both sides of the chops. Let rest at room temperature for 15 to 30 minutes.
2. Set the electric pressure cooker to Sauté/More setting. When hot, add the avocado oil.
3. Brown the lamb chops, about 2 minutes per side. (If they don't all fit in a single layer, brown them in batches.)
4. Transfer the chops to a plate. In the pot, combine the shallot, tomato paste, and broth. Cook for about a minute, scraping up the brown bits from the bottom. Hit Cancel.
5. Add the chops and any accumulated juices back to the pot.
6. Close and lock the lid of the pressure cooker. Set the valve to sealing.
7. Cook on high pressure for 2 minutes.
8. When the cooking is complete, hit Cancel and quick release the pressure.
9. Once the pin drops, unlock and remove the lid.
10. Place the lamb chops on plates and serve immediately.

Per Serving (1 lamb chop)
calories: 233 | fat: 18g | protein: 15g | carbs: 1g | sugars: 1g | fiber: 0g | sodium: 450mg

Zoodles Carbonara

Prep time: 10 minutes | Cook time: 25 minutes | Serves 4

6 slices bacon, cut into pieces
1 red onion, finely chopped
3 zucchini, cut into noodles
1 cup peas
½ teaspoon sea salt
3 garlic cloves, minced
3 large eggs, beaten
1 tablespoon heavy cream
Pinch red pepper flakes
½ cup grated Parmesan cheese (optional, for garnish)

1. In a large skillet over medium-high heat, cook the bacon until browned, about 5 minutes. With a slotted spoon, transfer the bacon to a plate.
2. Add the onion to the bacon fat in the pan and cook, stirring, until soft, 3 to 5 minutes. Add the zucchini, peas, and salt. Cook, stirring, until the zucchini softens, about 3 minutes. Add the garlic and cook, stirring constantly, for 5 minutes.
3. In a small bowl, whisk together the eggs, cream, and red pepper flakes. Add to the vegetables.
4. Remove the pan from the stove top and stir for 3 minutes, allowing the heat of the pan to cook the eggs without setting them.
5. Return the bacon to the pan and stir to mix.
6. Serve topped with Parmesan cheese, if desired.

Per Serving

calories: 326 | fat: 24g | protein: 14g | carbs: 15g | sugars: 2g | fiber: 4g | sodium: 555mg

Asian Grilled Beef Salad

Prep time: 15 minutes | Cook time: 15 minutes | Serves 4

Dressing:
¼ cup freshly squeezed lime juice
1 tablespoon low-sodium tamari or gluten-free soy sauce
1 tablespoon extra-virgin olive oil
1 garlic clove, minced
1 teaspoon honey
¼ teaspoon red pepper flakes

Salad:
1 pound (454 g) grass-fed flank steak
¼ teaspoon salt
Pinch freshly ground black pepper
6 cups chopped leaf lettuce
1 cucumber, halved lengthwise and thinly cut into half moons
½ small red onion, sliced
1 carrot, cut into ribbons
¼ cup chopped fresh cilantro

Make the Dressing
1. In a small bowl, whisk together the lime juice, tamari, olive oil, garlic, honey, and red pepper flakes. Set aside.

Make the Salad
1. Season the beef on both sides with the salt and pepper.
2. Heat a skillet over high heat until hot. Cook the beef for 3 to 6 minutes per side, depending on preferred doneness. Set aside, tented with aluminum foil, for 10 minutes.
3. In a large bowl, toss the lettuce, cucumber, onion, carrot, and cilantro.
4. Slice the beef thinly against the grain and transfer to the salad bowl.
5. Drizzle with the dressing and toss. Serve.

Per Serving

calories: 231 | fat: 10g | protein: 26g | carbs: 10g | sugars: 4g | fiber: 2g | sodium: 349mg

Pork Tenderloin Roast with Mango Glaze

Prep time: 10 minutes | Cook time: 20 minutes | Serves 4

1 pound (454 g) boneless pork tenderloin, trimmed of fat
1 teaspoon chopped fresh rosemary
1 teaspoon chopped fresh thyme
¼ teaspoon salt, divided
¼ teaspoon freshly ground black pepper, divided
1 teaspoon extra-virgin olive oil
1 tablespoon honey
2 tablespoons white wine vinegar
2 tablespoons dry cooking wine
1 tablespoon minced fresh ginger
1 cup diced mango

1. Preheat the oven to 400°F (205°C).
2. Season the tenderloin with the rosemary, thyme, ⅛ teaspoon of salt, and ⅛ teaspoon of pepper.
3. Heat the olive oil in an oven-safe skillet over medium-high heat, and sear the tenderloin until browned on all sides, about 5 minutes total.
4. Transfer the skillet to the oven and roast for 12 to 15 minutes until the pork is cooked through, the juices run clear, and the internal temperature reaches 145°F (63°C). Transfer to a cutting board to rest for 5 minutes.
5. In a small bowl, combine the honey, vinegar, cooking wine, and ginger. In to the same skillet, pour the honey mixture and simmer for 1 minute. Add the mango and toss to coat. Transfer to a blender and purée until smooth. Season with the remaining ⅛ teaspoon of salt and ⅛ teaspoon of pepper.
6. Slice the pork into rounds and serve with the mango sauce.

Per Serving
calories: 182 | fat: 4g | protein: 24g | carbs: 12g | sugars: 10g | fiber: 1g | sodium: 240mg

Cheeseburger and Cauliflower Wraps

Prep time: 5 minutes | Cook time: 20 minutes | Serves 4

Avocado oil cooking spray
½ cup chopped white onion
1 cup chopped portobello mushrooms
1 pound (454 g) 93% lean ground beef
½ teaspoon garlic powder
Pinch salt
1 (10-ounce / 283-g) bag frozen cauliflower rice
12 iceberg lettuce leaves
¾ cup shredded Cheddar cheese

1. Heat a large skillet over medium heat. When hot, coat the cooking surface with cooking spray and add the onion and mushrooms. Cook for 5 minutes, stirring occasionally.
2. Add the beef, garlic powder, and salt, stirring and breaking apart the meat as needed. Cook for 5 minutes.
3. Stir in the frozen cauliflower rice and increase the heat to medium-high. Cook for 5 minutes more, or until the water evaporates.
4. For each portion, use three lettuce leaves. Spoon one-quarter of the filling onto the lettuce leaves, and top with one-quarter of the cheese. Then, working from the side closest to you, roll up the lettuce to close the wrap. Repeat with the remaining lettuce leaves and filling.

Per Serving
calories: 288 | fat: 15g | protein: 31g | carbs: 7g | sugars: 4g | fiber: 3g | sodium: 264mg

Lamb and Vegetable Stew

Prep time: 10 minutes | Cook time: 3 to 6 hours | Serves 6

1 pound (454 g) boneless lamb stew meat
1 pound (454 g) turnips, peeled and chopped
1 fennel bulb, trimmed and thinly sliced
10 ounces (283 g) mushrooms, sliced
1 onion, diced
3 garlic cloves, minced
2 cups low-sodium chicken broth
2 tablespoons tomato paste
¼ cup dry red wine (optional)
1 teaspoon chopped fresh thyme
½ teaspoon salt
¼ teaspoon freshly ground black pepper
Chopped fresh parsley, for garnish

1. In a slow cooker, combine the lamb, turnips, fennel, mushrooms, onion, garlic, chicken broth, tomato paste, red wine (if using), thyme, salt, and pepper.
2. Cover and cook on high for 3 hours or on low for 6 hours. When the meat is tender and falling apart, garnish with parsley and serve.
3. If you don't have a slow cooker, in a large pot, heat 2 teaspoons of olive oil over medium heat, and sear the lamb on all sides. Remove from the pot and set aside. Add the turnips, fennel, mushrooms, onion, and garlic to the pot, and cook for 3 to 4 minutes until the vegetables begin to soften. Add the chicken broth, tomato paste, red wine (if using), thyme, salt, pepper, and browned lamb. Bring to a boil, then reduce the heat to low. Simmer for 1½ to 2 hours until the meat is tender. Garnish with parsley and serve.

Per Serving
calories: 303 | fat: 7g | protein: 32g | carbs: 27g | sugars: 7g | fiber: 4g | sodium: 310mg

Corned Beef and Cabbage Soup

Prep time: 15 minutes | Cook time: 26 minutes | Serves 4

2 tablespoons avocado oil
1 small onion, chopped
3 celery stalks, chopped
3 medium carrots, chopped
¼ teaspoon allspice
4 cups chicken bone broth, vegetable broth, low-sodium
store-bought beef broth, or water
4 cups sliced green cabbage (about ⅓ medium head)
¾ cup pearled barley
4 ounces (113 g) cooked corned beef, cut into thin strips or chunks
Freshly ground black pepper, to taste

1. Set the electric pressure cooker to the Sauté setting. When the pot is hot, pour in the avocado oil.
2. Sauté the onion, celery, and carrots for 3 to 5 minutes or until the vegetables begin to soften. Stir in the allspice. Hit Cancel.
3. Stir in the broth, cabbage, and barley.
4. Close and lock the lid of the pressure cooker. Set the valve to sealing.
5. Cook on high pressure for 20 minutes.
6. When the cooking is complete, allow the pressure to release naturally for 10 minutes, then quick release any remaining pressure. Hit Cancel.
7. Once the pin drops, unlock and remove the lid.
8. Stir in the corned beef, season with pepper, and replace the lid. Let the soup sit for about 5 minutes to let the corned beef warm up.
9. Spoon into serving bowls and serve.

Per Serving (1¼ cups)
calories: 321 | fat: 13g | protein: 11g | carbs: 42g | sugars: 7g | fiber: 11g | sodium: 412mg

5-Ingredient Mexican Lasagna

Prep time: 15 minutes | Cook time: 15 minutes | Serves 4

Nonstick cooking spray
½ (15-ounce / 425-g) can light red kidney beans, rinsed and drained
4 (6-inch) gluten-free corn tortillas
1½ cups cooked shredded beef, pork, or chicken
1⅓ cups salsa
1⅓ cups shredded Mexican cheese blend

1. Spray a 6-inch springform pan with nonstick spray. Wrap the bottom in foil.
2. In a medium bowl, mash the beans with a fork.
3. Place 1 tortilla in the bottom of the pan. Add about ⅓ of the beans, ½ cup of meat, ⅓ cup of salsa, and ⅓ cup of cheese. Press down. Repeat for 2 more layers. Add the remaining tortilla and press down. Top with the remaining salsa and cheese. There are no beans or meat on the top layer.
4. Tear off a piece of foil big enough to cover the pan, and spray it with nonstick spray. Line the pan with the foil, sprayed-side down.
5. Pour 1 cup of water into the electric pressure cooker.
6. Place the pan on the wire rack and carefully lower it into the pot. Close and lock the lid of the pressure cooker. Set the valve to sealing.
7. Cook on high pressure for 15 minutes.
8. When the cooking is complete, hit Cancel. Allow the pressure to release naturally for 10 minutes, then quick release any remaining pressure.
9. Once the pin drops, unlock and remove the lid.
10. Using the handles of the wire rack, carefully remove the pan from the pot. Let the lasagna sit for 5 minutes. Carefully remove the ring.
11. Slice into quarters and serve.

Per Serving
calories: 395 | fat: 16g | protein: 30g | carbs: 34g | sugars: 5g | fiber: 9g | sodium: 1140mg

Pork Chop Diane

Prep time: 10 minutes | Cook time: 20 minutes | Serves 4

¼ cup low-sodium chicken broth
1 tablespoon freshly squeezed lemon juice
2 teaspoons Worcestershire sauce
2 teaspoons Dijon mustard
4 (5-ounce / 142-g) boneless pork top loin chops, about 1 inch thick
Sea salt and freshly ground black pepper, to taste
1 teaspoon extra-virgin olive oil
1 teaspoon lemon zest
1 teaspoon butter
2 teaspoons chopped fresh chives

1. In a small bowl, stir together the chicken broth, lemon juice, Worcestershire sauce, and Dijon mustard and set it aside.
2. Season the pork chops lightly with salt and pepper.
3. Place a large skillet over medium-high heat and add the olive oil.
4. Cook the pork chops, turning once, until they are no longer pink, about 8 minutes per side.
5. Transfer the chops to a plate and set it aside.
6. Pour the broth mixture into the skillet and cook until warmed through and thickened, about 2 minutes.
7. Whisk in the lemon zest, butter, and chives.
8. Serve the chops with a generous spoonful of sauce.

Per Serving
calories: 200 | fat: 8g | protein: 30g | carbs: 1g | sugars: 1g | fiber: 0g | sodium: 394mg

Pork Chops with Red Cabbage and Apples

Prep time: 15 minutes | Cook time: 30 minutes | Serves 4

¼ cup apple cider vinegar
2 tablespoons granulated sweetener
4 (4-ounce / 113-g) pork chops, about 1 inch thick
Sea salt and freshly ground black pepper, to taste

1 tablespoon extra-virgin olive oil
½ red cabbage, finely shredded
1 sweet onion, thinly sliced
1 apple, peeled, cored, and sliced
1 teaspoon chopped fresh thyme

1. In a small bowl, whisk together the vinegar and sweetener. Set it aside.
2. Season the pork with salt and pepper.
3. Place a large skillet over medium-high heat and add the olive oil.
4. Cook the pork chops until no longer pink, turning once, about 8 minutes per side.
5. Transfer the chops to a plate and set aside.
6. Add the cabbage and onion to the skillet and sauté until the vegetables have softened, about 5 minutes.
7. Add the vinegar mixture and the apple slices to the skillet and bring the mixture to a boil.
8. Reduce the heat to low and simmer, covered, for 5 additional minutes.
9. Return the pork chops to the skillet, along with any accumulated juices and thyme, cover, and cook for 5 more minutes.

Per Serving
calories: 223 | fat: 8g | protein: 26g | carbs: 12g | sugars: 8g | fiber: 3g | sodium: 292mg

Orange-Marinated Pork Tenderloin

Prep time: 10 minutes | Cook time: 30 minutes | Serves 4

¼ cup freshly squeezed orange juice
2 teaspoons orange zest
2 teaspoons minced garlic
1 teaspoon low-sodium soy sauce

1 teaspoon grated fresh ginger
1 teaspoon honey
1½ pounds (680 g) pork tenderloin roast, trimmed of fat
1 tablespoon extra-virgin olive oil

1. In a small bowl, whisk together the orange juice, zest, garlic, soy sauce, ginger, and honey.
2. Pour the marinade into a resealable plastic bag and add the pork tenderloin.
3. Remove as much air as possible and seal the bag. Marinate the pork in the refrigerator, turning the bag a few times, for 2 hours.
4. Preheat the oven to 400ºF (205ºC).
5. Remove the tenderloin from the marinade and discard the marinade.
6. Place a large ovenproof skillet over medium-high heat and add the oil.
7. Sear the pork tenderloin on all sides, about 5 minutes in total.
8. Transfer the skillet to the oven and roast the pork until just cooked through, about 25 minutes.
9. Let the meat stand for 10 minutes before serving.

Per Serving
calories: 228 | fat: 9g | protein: 34g | carbs: 4g | sugars: 3g | fiber: 0g | sodium: 486mg

Roasted Beef with Peppercorn Sauce

Prep time: 10 minutes | Cook time: 1 hour 40 minutes | Serves 4

1½ pounds (680 g) top rump beef roast
Sea salt and freshly ground black pepper, to taste
3 teaspoons extra-virgin olive oil, divided
3 shallots, minced
2 teaspoons minced garlic
1 tablespoon green peppercorns
2 tablespoons dry sherry
2 tablespoons all-purpose flour
1 cup sodium-free beef broth

1. Heat the oven to 300ºF (150ºC).
2. Season the roast with salt and pepper.
3. Place a large skillet over medium-high heat and add 2 teaspoons of olive oil.
4. Brown the beef on all sides, about 10 minutes in total, and transfer the roast to a baking dish.
5. Roast until desired doneness, about 1½ hours for medium. When the roast has been in the oven for 1 hour, start the sauce.
6. In a medium saucepan over medium-high heat, sauté the shallots in the remaining 1 teaspoon of olive oil until translucent, about 4 minutes.
7. Stir in the garlic and peppercorns, and cook for another minute. Whisk in the sherry to deglaze the pan.
8. Whisk in the flour to form a thick paste, cooking for 1 minute and stirring constantly.
9. Pour in the beef broth and whisk until the sauce is thick and glossy, about 4 minutes. Season the sauce with salt and pepper.
10. Serve the beef with a generous spoonful of sauce.

Per Serving

calories: 330 | fat: 18g | protein: 36g | carbs: 4g | sugars: 1g | fiber: 0g | sodium: 207mg

Coffee-and-Herb-Marinated Steak

Prep time: 10 minutes | Cook time: 10 minutes | Serves 4

¼ cup whole coffee beans
2 teaspoons minced garlic
2 teaspoons chopped fresh rosemary
2 teaspoons chopped fresh thyme
1 teaspoon freshly ground black pepper
2 tablespoons apple cider vinegar
2 tablespoons extra-virgin olive oil
1 pound (454 g) flank steak, trimmed of visible fat

1. Place the coffee beans, garlic, rosemary, thyme, and black pepper in a coffee grinder or food processor and pulse until coarsely ground.
2. Transfer the coffee mixture to a resealable plastic bag and add the vinegar and oil. Shake to combine.
3. Add the flank steak and squeeze the excess air out of the bag. Seal it. Marinate the steak in the refrigerator for at least 2 hours, occasionally turning the bag over.
4. Preheat the broiler. Line a baking sheet with aluminum foil.
5. Take the steak out of the bowl and discard the marinade.
6. Place the steak on the baking sheet and broil until it is done to your liking, about 5 minutes per side for medium.
7. Let the steak rest for 10 minutes before slicing it thinly on a bias.
8. Serve with a mixed green salad or your favorite side dish.

Per Serving

calories: 313 | fat: 20g | protein: 31g | carbs: 0g | sugars: 0g | fiber: 0g | sodium: 79mg

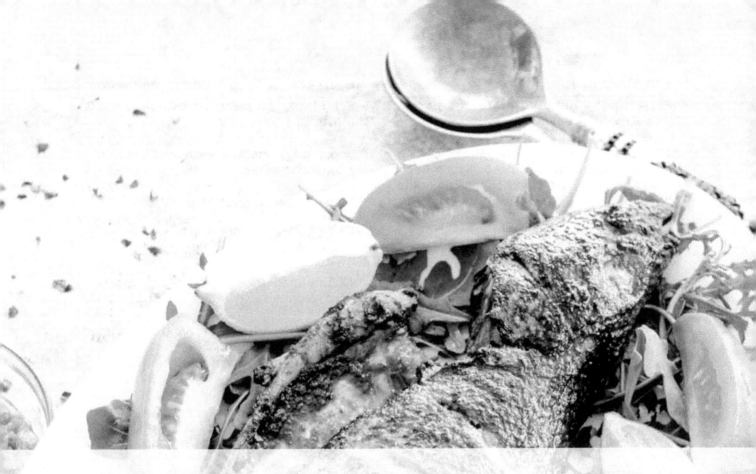
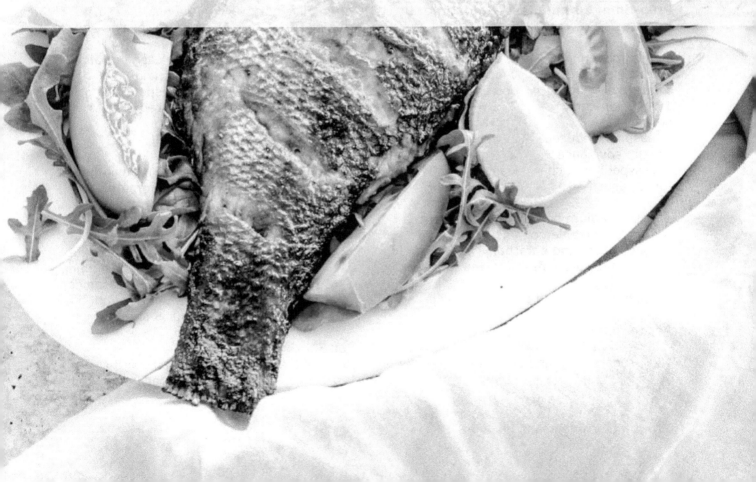

Chapter 8 Fish and Seafood

Tomato Bun Tuna Melts

Prep time: 5 minutes | Cook time: 5 minutes | Serves 2

1 (5-ounce / 142-g) can chunk light tuna packed in water, drained
2 tablespoons plain nonfat Greek yogurt
2 teaspoons freshly squeezed lemon juice
2 tablespoons finely chopped celery
1 tablespoon finely chopped red onion
Pinch cayenne pepper
1 large tomato, cut into ¾-inch-thick rounds
½ cup shredded Cheddar cheese

1. Preheat the broiler to high.
2. In a medium bowl, combine the tuna, yogurt, lemon juice, celery, red onion, and cayenne pepper. Stir well.
3. Arrange the tomato slices on a baking sheet. Top each with some tuna salad and Cheddar cheese.
4. Broil for 3 to 4 minutes until the cheese is melted and bubbly. Serve.

Per Serving

calories: 243 | fat: 10g | protein: 30g | carbs: 7g | sugars: 2g | fiber: 1g | sodium: 444mg

Curried Tuna Salad Lettuce Wraps

Prep time: 10 minutes | Cook time: 0 minutes | Serves 2

⅓ cup mayonnaise
1 tablespoon freshly squeezed lemon juice
1 teaspoon curry powder
1 teaspoon reduced-sodium soy sauce
½ teaspoon sriracha (or to taste)
½ cup canned water chestnuts, drained and chopped
2 (2.6-ounce / 74-g) package tuna packed in water, drained
2 large butter lettuce leaves

1. In a medium bowl, whisk together the mayonnaise, lemon juice, curry powder, soy sauce, and sriracha.
2. Add the water chestnuts and tuna. Stir to combine.
3. Serve wrapped in the lettuce leaves.

Per Serving

calories: 271 | fat: 14g | protein: 19g | carbs: 18g | sugars: 1g | fiber: 3g | sodium: 627mg

Corn and Shrimp Salad in Avocado

Prep time: 10 minutes | Cook time: 0 minutes | Serves 2

¼ cup mayonnaise
1 teaspoon sriracha (or to taste)
½ teaspoon lemon zest
¼ teaspoon sea salt
4 ounces (113 g)
cooked baby shrimp
½ cup cooked and cooled corn kernels
½ red bell pepper, seeded and chopped
1 avocado, halved lengthwise

1. In a medium bowl, combine the mayonnaise, sriracha, lemon zest, and salt.
2. Add the shrimp, corn, and bell pepper. Mix to combine.
3. Spoon the mixture into the avocado halves.

Per Serving

calories: 326 | fat: 21g | protein: 15g | carbs: 25g | sugars: 1g | fiber: 7g | sodium: 538mg

Cioppino

Prep time: 10 minutes | Cook time: 20 minutes | Serves 4

2 tablespoons extra-virgin olive oil
1 onion, finely chopped
1 garlic clove, minced
½ cup dry white wine
1 (14-ounce / 397-g) can tomato sauce
8 ounces (227 g) cod, pin bones removed,
cut into 1-inch pieces
8 ounces (227 g) shrimp, peeled and deveined
1 tablespoon Italian seasoning
½ teaspoon sea salt
Pinch red pepper flakes

1. In a large skillet over medium-high heat, heat the olive oil until it shimmers. Add the onion and cook, stirring occasionally, for 3 minutes. Add the garlic and cook, stirring constantly, for 30 seconds. Add the wine and cook, stirring, for 1 minute.
2. Add the tomato sauce. Bring to a simmer. Stir in the cod, shrimp, Italian seasoning, salt, and pepper flakes. Simmer until the fish is just opaque, about 5 minutes.

Per Serving

calories: 243 | fat: 8g | protein: 23g | carbs: 11g | sugars: 7g | fiber: 2g | sodium: 271mg

Tuna Patties

Prep time: 5 minutes | Cook time: 10 minutes | Serves 4

1 pound (454 g) canned tuna, drained
1 cup whole-wheat bread crumbs
2 large eggs, beaten
½ onion, grated
1 tablespoon chopped
fresh dill
Juice and zest of 1 lemon
3 tablespoons extra-virgin olive oil
½ cup tartar sauce, for serving

1. In a large bowl, combine the tuna, bread crumbs, eggs, onion, dill, and lemon juice and zest. Form the mixture into 4 patties and chill for 10 minutes.
2. In a large nonstick skillet over medium-high heat, heat the olive oil until it shimmers. Add the patties and cook until browned on both sides, 4 to 5 minutes per side.
3. Serve topped with the tartar sauce.

Per Serving

calories: 530 | fat: 34g | protein: 35g | carbs: 18g | sugars: 3g | fiber: 2g | sodium: 674mg

Honey Mustard Roasted Salmon

Prep time: 5 minutes | Cook time: 20 minutes | Serves 4

Nonstick cooking spray
2 tablespoons whole-grain mustard
1 tablespoon honey
2 garlic cloves,
minced
¼ teaspoon salt
¼ teaspoon freshly ground black pepper
1 pound (454 g) salmon fillet

1. Preheat the oven to 425ºF (220ºC). Spray a baking sheet with nonstick cooking spray.
2. In a small bowl, whisk together the mustard, honey, garlic, salt, and pepper.
3. Place the salmon fillet on the prepared baking sheet, skin-side down. Spoon the sauce onto the salmon and spread evenly.
4. Roast for 15 to 20 minutes, depending on the thickness of the fillet, until the flesh flakes easily.

Per Serving

calories: 186 | fat: 7g | protein: 23g | carbs: 6g | sugars: 4g | fiber: 0g | sodium: 312mg

Cod with Mango Salsa

Prep time: 10 minutes | Cook time: 10 minutes | Serves 4

1 pound (454 g) cod, cut into 4 fillets, pin bones removed
2 tablespoons extra-virgin olive oil
¾ teaspoon sea salt, divided
1 mango, pitted, peeled, and cut into
cubes
¼ cup chopped cilantro
½ red onion, finely chopped
1 jalapeño, seeded and finely chopped
1 garlic clove, minced
Juice of 1 lime

1. Preheat the oven broiler on high.
2. On a rimmed baking sheet, brush the cod with the olive oil and season with ½ teaspoon of the salt. Broil until the fish is opaque, 5 to 10 minutes.
3. Meanwhile, in a small bowl, combine the mango, cilantro, onion, jalapeño, garlic, lime juice, and remaining ¼ teaspoon of salt.
4. Serve the cod with the salsa spooned over the top.

Per Serving

calories: 197 | fat: 8g | protein: 21g | carbs: 13g | sugars: 12g | fiber: 2g | sodium: 354mg

Avocado-Tuna with Croutons

Prep time: 10 minutes | Cook time: 0 minutes | Serves 3

2 (5-ounce / 142-g) cans chunk-light tuna, drained
2 tablespoons low-fat mayonnaise
½ teaspoon freshly
ground black pepper
3 avocados, halved and pitted
6 tablespoons packaged croutons

1. In a medium bowl, combine the tuna, mayonnaise, and pepper, and mix well.
2. Top the avocados with the tuna mixture and croutons.

Per Serving

calories: 428 | fat: 29g | protein: 28g | carbs: 19g | sugars: 1g | fiber: 12g | sodium: 167mg

Air Fryer Fish Fry

Prep time: 5 minutes | Cook time: 15 minutes | Serves 4

2 cups low-fat buttermilk
½ teaspoon garlic powder
½ teaspoon onion powder
4 (4-ounce / 113-g) flounder fillets
½ cup plain yellow cornmeal
½ cup chickpea flour
¼ teaspoon cayenne pepper
Freshly ground black pepper, to taste

1. In a large bowl, combine the buttermilk, garlic powder, and onion powder.
2. Add the flounder, turning until well coated, and set aside to marinate for 20 minutes.
3. In a shallow bowl, stir the cornmeal, chickpea flour, cayenne, and pepper together.
4. Dredge the fillets in the meal mixture, turning until well coated. Place in the basket of an air fryer.
5. Set the air fryer to 380ºF (193ºC), close, and cook for 12 minutes.

Per Serving
calories: 229 | fat: 6g | protein: 28g | carbs: 16g | sugars: 7g | fiber: 2g | sodium: 241mg

Ginger-Garlic Fish in Parchment

Prep time: 10 minutes | Cook time: 15 minutes | Serves 4

1 chard bunch, stemmed, leaves and stems cut into thin strips
1 red bell pepper, seeded and cut into strips
1 pound (454 g) cod fillets cut into 4 pieces
1 tablespoon grated fresh ginger
3 garlic cloves, minced
2 tablespoons white wine vinegar
2 tablespoons low-sodium tamari or gluten-free soy sauce
1 tablespoon honey

1. Preheat the oven to 425ºF (220ºC).
2. Cut four pieces of parchment paper, each about 16 inches wide. Lay the four pieces out on a large workspace.
3. On each piece of paper, arrange a small pile of chard leaves and stems, topped by several strips of bell pepper. Top with a piece of cod.
4. In a small bowl, mix the ginger, garlic, vinegar, tamari, and honey. Top each piece of fish with one-fourth of the mixture.
5. Fold the parchment paper over so the edges overlap. Fold the edges over several times to secure the fish in the packets. Carefully place the packets on a large baking sheet.
6. Bake for 12 minutes. Carefully open the packets, allowing steam to escape, and serve.

Per Serving
calories: 118 | fat: 1g | protein: 19g | carbs: 9g | sugars: 6g | fiber: 1g | sodium: 715mg

Whole Veggie-Stuffed Trout

Prep time: 10 minutes | Cook time: 25 minutes | Serves 2

Nonstick cooking spray
2 (8-ounce / 227-g) whole trout fillets, dressed (cleaned but with bones and skin intact)
1 tablespoon extra-virgin olive oil
¼ teaspoon salt
⅛ teaspoon freshly ground black pepper
½ red bell pepper, seeded and thinly sliced
1 small onion, thinly sliced
2 or 3 shiitake mushrooms, sliced
1 poblano pepper, seeded and thinly sliced
1 lemon, sliced

1. Preheat the oven to 425ºF (220ºC). Spray a baking sheet with nonstick cooking spray.
2. Rub both trout, inside and out, with the olive oil, then season with the salt and pepper.
3. In a large bowl, combine the bell pepper, onion, mushrooms, and poblano pepper. Stuff half of this mixture into the cavity of each fish. Top the mixture with 2 or 3 lemon slices inside each fish.
4. Arrange the fish on the prepared baking sheet side by side and roast for 25 minutes until the fish is cooked through and the vegetables are tender.

Per Serving
calories: 452 | fat: 22g | protein: 49g | carbs: 14g | sugars: 2g | fiber: 3g | sodium: 357mg

Lemon Pepper Salmon

Prep time: 5 minutes | Cook time: 20 minutes | Serves 4

Nonstick cooking spray
½ teaspoon freshly ground black pepper
¼ teaspoon salt
Zest and juice of ½

lemon
¼ teaspoon dried thyme
1 pound (454 g) salmon fillet

1. Preheat the oven to 425ºF (220ºC). Spray a baking sheet with nonstick cooking spray.
2. In a small bowl, combine the pepper, salt, lemon zest and juice, and thyme. Stir to combine.
3. Place the salmon on the prepared baking sheet, skin-side down. Spread the seasoning mixture evenly over the fillet.
4. Bake for 15 to 20 minutes, depending on the thickness of the fillet, until the flesh flakes easily.

Per Serving
calories: 163 | fat: 7g | protein: 23g | carbs: 1g | sugars: 0g | fiber: 0g | sodium: 167mg

Honey Ginger Glazed Salmon with Broccoli

Prep time: 10 minutes | Cook time: 15 minutes | Serves 4

Nonstick cooking spray
1 tablespoon low-sodium tamari or gluten-free soy sauce
Juice of 1 lemon
1 tablespoon honey
1 (1-inch) piece fresh ginger, grated
1 garlic clove, minced

1 pound (454 g) salmon fillet
¼ teaspoon salt, divided
⅛ teaspoon freshly ground black pepper
2 broccoli heads, cut into florets
1 tablespoon extra-virgin olive oil

1. Preheat the oven to 400ºF (205ºC). Spray a baking sheet with nonstick cooking spray.
2. In a small bowl, mix the tamari, lemon juice, honey, ginger, and garlic. Set aside.
3. Place the salmon skin-side down on the prepared baking sheet. Season with ⅛ teaspoon of salt and the pepper.
4. In a large mixing bowl, toss the broccoli and olive oil. Season with the remaining ⅛ teaspoon of salt. Arrange in a single layer on the baking sheet next to the salmon. Bake for 15 to 20 minutes until the salmon flakes easily with a fork and the broccoli is fork-tender.
5. In a small pan over medium heat, bring the tamari-ginger mixture to a simmer and cook for 1 to 2 minutes until it just begins to thicken.
6. Drizzle the sauce over the salmon and serve.

Per Serving
calories: 238 | fat: 11g | protein: 25g | carbs: 11g | sugars: 6g | fiber: 2g | sodium: 334mg

Herb-Crusted Halibut

Prep time: 10 minutes | Cook time: 20 minutes | Serves 4

4 (5-ounce / 142-g) halibut fillets
Extra-virgin olive oil, for brushing
½ cup coarsely ground unsalted pistachios
1 tablespoon chopped

fresh parsley
1 teaspoon chopped fresh thyme
1 teaspoon chopped fresh basil
Pinch sea salt
Pinch freshly ground black pepper

1. Preheat the oven to 350ºF (180ºC).
2. Line a baking sheet with parchment paper.
3. Pat the halibut fillets dry with a paper towel and place them on the baking sheet.
4. Brush the halibut generously with olive oil.
5. In a small bowl, stir together the pistachios, parsley, thyme, basil, salt, and pepper.
6. Spoon the nut and herb mixture evenly on the fish, spreading it out so the tops of the fillets are covered.
7. Bake the halibut until it flakes when pressed with a fork, about 20 minutes.
8. Serve immediately.

Per Serving
calories: 262 | fat: 11g | protein: 32g | carbs: 4g | sugars: 1g | fiber: 2g | sodium: 77mg

Open-Faced Tuna Melts

Prep time: 5 minutes | Cook time: 5 minutes | Serves 3

3 English muffins, 100% whole-wheat
2 (5-ounce / 142-g) cans chunk-light tuna, drained
3 tablespoons plain
low-fat Greek yogurt
½ teaspoon freshly ground black pepper
¾ cup shredded Cheddar cheese

1. If your broiler is in the top of your oven, place the oven rack in the center position. Turn the broiler on high.
2. Split the English muffins, if necessary, and toast them in the toaster.
3. Meanwhile, in a medium bowl, mix the tuna, yogurt, and pepper.
4. Place the muffin halves on a baking sheet, and spoon one-sixth of the tuna mixture and 2 tablespoons of Cheddar cheese on top of each half. Broil for 2 minutes or until the cheese melts.

Per Serving

calories: 392 | fat: 13g | protein: 40g | carbs: 28g | sugars: 6g | fiber: 5g | sodium: 474mg

Shrimp Stir-Fry

Prep time: 5 minutes | Cook time: 15 minutes | Serves 4

Sauce:
½ cup water
2½ tablespoons low-sodium soy sauce
2 tablespoons honey
1 tablespoon rice vinegar
¼ teaspoon garlic powder
Pinch ground ginger
1 tablespoon cornstarch
Stir-Fry:
8 cups frozen vegetable stir-fry mix
2 tablespoons sesame oil
40 medium fresh shrimp, peeled and deveined

Make the Sauce
1. In a small saucepan, whisk together the water, soy sauce, honey, rice vinegar, garlic powder, and ginger. Add the cornstarch and whisk until fully incorporated.
2. Bring the sauce to a boil over medium heat. Boil for 1 minute to thicken. Remove the sauce from the heat and set aside.

Make the Stir-Fry
1. Heat a large saucepan over medium-high heat. When hot, put the vegetable stir-fry mix into the pan, and cook for 7 to 10 minutes, stirring occasionally until the water completely evaporates.
2. Reduce the heat to medium-low, add the oil and shrimp, and stir. Cook for about 3 minutes, or until the shrimp are pink and opaque.
3. Add the sauce to the shrimp and vegetables and stir to coat. Cook for 2 minutes more.

Per Serving

calories: 297 | fat: 17g | protein: 24g | carbs: 14g | sugars: 9g | fiber: 2g | sodium: 454mg

Fish Tacos

Prep time: 5 minutes | Cook time: 10 minutes | Serves 4

Tacos:
2 tablespoons extra-virgin olive oil
4 (6-ounce / 170-g) cod fillets
8 (10-inch) yellow corn tortillas
2 cups packaged shredded cabbage
¼ cup chopped fresh cilantro
4 lime wedges
Sauce:
½ cup plain low-fat Greek yogurt
⅓ cup low-fat mayonnaise
½ teaspoon garlic powder
½ teaspoon ground cumin

Make the Tacos
1. Heat a medium skillet over medium-low heat. When hot, pour the oil into the skillet, then add the fish and cover. Cook for 4 minutes, then flip and cook for 4 minutes more.
2. Top each tortilla with one-eighth of the cabbage, sauce, cilantro, and fish. Finish each taco with a squeeze of lime.
Make the Sauce
1. In a small bowl, whisk together the yogurt, mayonnaise, garlic powder, and cumin.

Per Serving

calories: 373 | fat: 13g | protein: 36g | carbs: 30g | sugars: 4g | fiber: 4g | sodium: 342mg

Creamy Cod with Asparagus

Prep time: 5 minutes | Cook time: 15 minutes | Serves 4

½ cup uncooked brown rice or quinoa
4 (4-ounce / 113-g) cod fillets
¼ teaspoon salt
¼ teaspoon freshly ground black pepper
½ teaspoon garlic powder, divided
24 asparagus spears
Avocado oil cooking spray
1 cup half-and-half

1. Cook the rice according to the package instructions.
2. Meanwhile, season both sides of the cod fillets with the salt, pepper, and ¼ teaspoon of garlic powder.
3. Cut the bottom 1½ inches from the asparagus.
4. Heat a large pan over medium-low heat. When hot, coat the cooking surface with cooking spray, and arrange the cod and asparagus in a single layer.
5. Cover and cook for 8 minutes.
6. Add the half-and-half and the remaining ¼ teaspoon of garlic powder and stir. Increase the heat to high and simmer for 2 minutes.
7. Divide the rice, cod, and asparagus into four equal portions.

Per Serving

calories: 257 | fat: 8g | protein: 25g | carbs: 23g | sugars: 4g | fiber: 5g | sodium: 411mg

Catfish with Corn and Pepper Relish

Prep time: 10 minutes | Cook time: 10 minutes | Serves 4

3 tablespoons extra-virgin olive oil, divided
4 (5-ounce / 142-g) catfish fillets
¼ teaspoon salt
¼ teaspoon freshly ground black pepper
1 (15-ounce / 425-g) can low-sodium black
beans, drained and rinsed
1 cup frozen corn
1 medium red bell pepper, diced
1 tablespoon apple cider vinegar
3 tablespoons chopped scallions

1. Use 1½ tablespoons of oil to coat both sides of the catfish fillets, then season the fillets with the salt and pepper.
2. Heat a small saucepan over medium-high heat. Put the remaining 1½ tablespoons of oil, beans, corn, bell pepper, and vinegar in the pan and stir. Cover and cook for 5 minutes.
3. Place the catfish fillets on top of the relish mixture and cover. Cook for 5 to 7 minutes.
4. Serve each catfish fillet with one-quarter of the relish and top with the scallions.

Per Serving

calories: 409 | fat: 21g | protein: 28g | carbs: 27g | sugars: 4g | fiber: 6g | sodium: 341mg

Lemon Salmon with Brussels Sprouts

Prep time: 5 minutes | Cook time: 20 minutes | Serves 4

Avocado oil cooking spray
20 Brussels sprouts, halved lengthwise
4 (4-ounce / 113-g) skinless salmon fillets
½ teaspoon garlic
powder
½ teaspoon freshly ground black pepper
¼ teaspoon salt
2 teaspoons freshly squeezed lemon juice

1. Heat a large skillet over medium-low heat. When hot, coat the cooking surface with cooking spray, and put the Brussels sprouts cut-side down in the skillet. Cover and cook for 5 minutes.
2. Meanwhile, season both sides of the salmon with the garlic powder, pepper, and salt.
3. Flip the Brussels sprouts, and move them to one side of the skillet. Add the salmon and cook, uncovered, for 4 to 6 minutes.
4. Check the Brussels sprouts. When they are tender, remove them from the skillet and set them aside.
5. Flip the salmon fillets. Cook for 4 to 6 more minutes, or until the salmon is opaque and flakes easily with a fork. Remove the salmon from the skillet, and let it rest for 5 minutes.
6. Divide the Brussels sprouts into four equal portions and add 1 salmon fillet to each portion. Sprinkle the lemon juice on top and serve.

Per Serving

calories: 193 | fat: 7g | protein: 25g | carbs: 10g | sugars: 2g | fiber: 4g | sodium: 222mg

Teriyaki Salmon

Prep time: 5 minutes | Cook time: 4 minutes | Serves 4

⅓ cup pineapple juice
⅓ cup reduced-sodium soy sauce
¼ cup water
2 tablespoons rice vinegar
1 tablespoon honey
1 garlic clove, minced

1 teaspoon peeled and grated fresh ginger
Pinch red pepper flakes
1 pound (454 g) salmon fillet, cut into 4 pieces

1. Preheat the oven broiler on high.
2. In a small bowl, whisk together the pineapple juice, soy sauce, water, vinegar, honey, garlic, ginger, and red pepper flakes.
3. Place the salmon pieces flesh-side down in the mixture for 5 minutes.
4. Place the salmon on a rimmed baking sheet, flesh-side up. Gently brush with any leftover sauce.
5. Broil until the salmon is opaque, 3 to 5 minutes.

Per Serving

calories: 202 | fat: 7g | protein: 24g | carbs: 9g | sugars: 7g | fiber: 0g | sodium: 752mg

Shrimp with Tomatoes and Feta

Prep time: 10 minutes | Cook time: 30 minutes | Serves 4

3 tomatoes, coarsely chopped
½ cup chopped sun-dried tomatoes
2 teaspoons minced garlic
2 teaspoons extra-virgin olive oil
1 teaspoon chopped fresh oregano

Freshly ground black pepper, to taste
1½ pounds (680 g) shrimp, peeled, deveined, tails removed
4 teaspoons freshly squeezed lemon juice
½ cup low-sodium feta cheese, crumbled

1. Heat the oven to 450°F (235°C).
2. In a medium bowl, toss the tomatoes, sun-dried tomatoes, garlic, oil, and oregano until well combined.
3. Season the mixture lightly with pepper.
4. Transfer the tomato mixture to a 9-by-13-inch glass baking dish.
5. Bake until softened, about 15 minutes.
6. Stir the shrimp and lemon juice into the hot tomato mixture and top evenly with the feta.
7. Bake until the shrimp are cooked through, about 15 minutes more.

Per Serving

calories: 306 | fat: 11g | protein: 39g | carbs: 12g | sugars: 5g | fiber: 3g | sodium: 502mg

Seared Scallops with Asparagus

Prep time: 10 minutes | Cook time: 15 minutes | Serves 4

3 teaspoons extra-virgin olive oil, divided
1 pound (454 g) asparagus, trimmed and cut into 2-inch segments
1 tablespoon butter
1 pound (454 g) sea

scallops
¼ cup dry white wine
Juice of 1 lemon
2 garlic cloves, minced
¼ teaspoon freshly ground black pepper

1. In a large skillet, heat 1½ teaspoons of oil over medium heat.
2. Add the asparagus and sauté for 5 to 6 minutes until just tender, stirring regularly. Remove from the skillet and cover with aluminum foil to keep warm.
3. Add the remaining 1½ teaspoons of oil and the butter to the skillet. When the butter is melted and sizzling, place the scallops in a single layer in the skillet. Cook for about 3 minutes on one side until nicely browned. Use tongs to gently loosen and flip the scallops, and cook on the other side for another 3 minutes until browned and cooked through. Remove and cover with foil to keep warm.
4. In the same skillet, combine the wine, lemon juice, garlic, and pepper. Bring to a simmer for 1 to 2 minutes, stirring to mix in any browned pieces left in the pan.
5. Return the asparagus and the cooked scallops to the skillet to coat with the sauce. Serve warm.

Per Serving

calories: 252 | fat: 7g | protein: 26g | carbs: 15g | sugars: 3g | fiber: 2g | sodium: 493mg

Spicy Citrus Sole

Prep time: 10 minutes | Cook time: 10 minutes | Serves 4

1 teaspoon chili powder
1 teaspoon garlic powder
½ teaspoon lime zest
½ teaspoon lemon zest
¼ teaspoon freshly ground black pepper

¼ teaspoon smoked paprika
Pinch sea salt
4 (6-ounce / 170-g) sole fillets, patted dry
1 tablespoon extra-virgin olive oil
2 teaspoons freshly squeezed lime juice

1. Preheat the oven to 450ºF (235ºC).
2. Line a baking sheet with aluminum foil and set it aside.
3. In a small bowl, stir together the chili powder, garlic powder, lime zest, lemon zest, pepper, paprika, and salt until well mixed.
4. Pat the fish fillets dry with paper towels, place them on the baking sheet, and rub them lightly all over with the spice mixture.
5. Drizzle the olive oil and lime juice on the top of the fish.
6. Bake until the fish flakes when pressed lightly with a fork, about 8 minutes. Serve immediately.

Per Serving
calories: 184 | fat: 5g | protein: 32g | carbs: 0g | sugars: 0g | fiber: 0g | sodium: 137mg

Haddock with Creamy Cucumber Sauce

Prep time: 10 minutes | Cook time: 10 minutes | Serves 4

¼ cup 2 percent plain Greek yogurt
½ English cucumber, grated, liquid squeezed out
½ scallion, white and green parts, finely chopped
2 teaspoons chopped

fresh mint
1 teaspoon honey
Sea salt, to taste
4 (5-ounce / 142-g) haddock fillets
Freshly ground black pepper, to taste
Nonstick cooking spray

1. In a small bowl, stir together the yogurt, cucumber, scallion, mint, honey, and a pinch of salt. Set it aside.

2. Pat the fish fillets dry with paper towels and season them lightly with salt and pepper.
3. Place a large skillet over medium-high heat and spray lightly with cooking spray.
4. Cook the haddock, turning once, until it is just cooked through, about 5 minutes per side.
5. Remove the fish from the heat and transfer to plates.
6. Serve topped with the cucumber sauce.

Per Serving
calories: 164 | fat: 2g | protein: 27g | carbs: 4g | sugars: 3g | fiber: 0g | sodium: 104mg

Baked Salmon with Lemon Sauce

Prep time: 10 minutes | Cook time: 15 minutes | Serves 4

4 (5-ounce / 142-g) salmon fillets
Sea salt and freshly ground black pepper, to taste
1 tablespoon extra-virgin olive oil
½ cup low-sodium vegetable broth

Juice and zest of 1 lemon
1 teaspoon chopped fresh thyme
½ cup fat-free sour cream
1 teaspoon honey
1 tablespoon chopped fresh chives

1. Preheat the oven to 400ºF (205ºC).
2. Season the salmon lightly on both sides with salt and pepper.
3. Place a large ovenproof skillet over medium-high heat and add the olive oil.
4. Sear the salmon fillets on both sides until golden, about 3 minutes per side.
5. Transfer the salmon to a baking dish and bake until it is just cooked through, about 10 minutes.
6. While the salmon is baking, whisk together the vegetable broth, lemon juice, zest, and thyme in a small saucepan over medium-high heat until the liquid reduces by about one-quarter, about 5 minutes.
7. Whisk in the sour cream and honey.
8. Stir in the chives and serve the sauce over the salmon.

Per Serving
calories: 310 | fat: 18g | protein: 29g | carbs: 6g | sugars: 2g | fiber: 0g | sodium: 129mg

Salmon Florentine

Prep time: 10 minutes | Cook time: 30 minutes | Serves 4

1 teaspoon extra-virgin olive oil
½ sweet onion, finely chopped
1 teaspoon minced garlic
3 cups baby spinach
1 cup kale, tough stems removed, torn

into 3-inch pieces
Sea salt and freshly ground black pepper, to taste
4 (5-ounce / 142-g) salmon fillets
Lemon wedges, for serving

1. Preheat the oven to 350ºF (180ºC).
2. Place a large skillet over medium-high heat and add the oil.
3. Sauté the onion and garlic until softened and translucent, about 3 minutes.
4. Add the spinach and kale and sauté until the greens wilt, about 5 minutes.
5. Remove the skillet from the heat and season the greens with salt and pepper.
6. Place the salmon fillets so they are nestled in the greens and partially covered by them. Bake the salmon until it is opaque, about 20 minutes.
7. Serve immediately with a squeeze of fresh lemon.

Per Serving

calories: 281 | fat: 16g | protein: 29g | carbs: 4g | sugars: 1g | fiber: 1g | sodium: 91mg

Halibut Roasted with Green Beans

Prep time: 10 minutes | Cook time: 15 minutes | Serves 4

1 pound (454 g) green beans, trimmed
2 red bell peppers, seeded and cut into strips
1 onion, sliced
Zest and juice of 2 lemons
3 garlic cloves, minced

2 tablespoons extra-virgin olive oil
1 teaspoon dried dill
1 teaspoon dried oregano
4 (4-ounce / 113-g) halibut fillets
½ teaspoon salt
¼ teaspoon freshly ground black pepper

1. Preheat the oven to 400ºF (205ºC). Line a baking sheet with parchment paper.
2. In a large bowl, toss the green beans, bell peppers, onion, lemon zest and juice, garlic, olive oil, dill, and oregano.

3. Use a slotted spoon to transfer the vegetables to the prepared baking sheet in a single layer, leaving the juice behind in the bowl.
4. Gently place the halibut fillets in the bowl, and coat in the juice. Transfer the fillets to the baking sheet, nestled between the vegetables, and drizzle them with any juice left in the bowl. Sprinkle the vegetables and halibut with the salt and pepper.
5. Bake for 15 to 20 minutes until the vegetables are just tender and the fish flakes apart easily.

Per Serving

calories: 234 | fat: 9g | protein: 24g | carbs: 16g | sugars: 8g | fiber: 5g | sodium: 349mg

Orange-Infused Scallops

Prep time: 10 minutes | Cook time: 10 minutes | Serves 4

2 pounds (907 g) sea scallops
Sea salt and freshly ground black pepper, to taste
2 tablespoons extra-virgin olive oil
1 tablespoon minced garlic

¼ cup freshly squeezed orange juice
1 teaspoon orange zest
2 teaspoons chopped fresh thyme, for garnish

1. Clean the scallops and pat them dry with paper towels, then season them lightly with salt and pepper.
2. Place a large skillet over medium-high heat and add the olive oil.
3. Sauté the garlic until it is softened and translucent, about 3 minutes.
4. Add the scallops to the skillet and cook until they are lightly seared and just cooked through, turning once, about 4 minutes per side.
5. Transfer the scallops to a plate, cover to keep warm, and set them aside.
6. Add the orange juice and zest to the skillet and stir to scrape up any cooked bits.
7. Spoon the sauce over the scallops and serve, garnished with the thyme.

Per Serving

calories: 267 | fat: 8g | protein: 38g | carbs: 8g | sugars: 1g | fiber: 0g | sodium: 361mg

Sole Piccata

Prep time: 10 minutes | Cook time: 20 minutes | Serves 4

1 teaspoon extra-virgin olive oil	2 tablespoons all-purpose flour
4 (5-ounce / 142-g) sole fillets, patted dry	2 cups low-sodium chicken broth
3 tablespoons butter	Juice and zest of ½ lemon
2 teaspoons minced garlic	2 tablespoons capers

1. Place a large skillet over medium-high heat and add the olive oil.
2. Pat the sole fillets dry with paper towels then pan-sear them until the fish flakes easily when tested with a fork, about 4 minutes on each side. Transfer the fish to a plate and set it aside.
3. Return the skillet to the stove and add the butter.
4. Sauté the garlic until translucent, about 3 minutes.
5. Whisk in the flour to make a thick paste and cook, stirring constantly, until the mixture is golden brown, about 2 minutes.
6. Whisk in the chicken broth, lemon juice, and lemon zest.
7. Cook until the sauce has thickened, about 4 minutes.
8. Stir in the capers and serve the sauce over the fish.

Per Serving
calories: 271 | fat: 13g | protein: 30g | carbs: 7g | sugars: 2g | fiber: 0g | sodium: 413mg

Lemon Butter Cod with Asparagus

Prep time: 5 minutes | Cook time: 15 minutes | Serves 4

½ cup uncooked brown rice or quinoa	¼ teaspoon garlic powder
4 (4-ounce / 113-g) cod fillets	24 asparagus spears
¼ teaspoon salt	2 tablespoons unsalted butter
¼ teaspoon freshly ground black pepper	1 tablespoon freshly squeezed lemon juice

1. Cook the rice according to the package instructions.
2. Meanwhile, season both sides of the cod fillets with the salt, pepper, and garlic powder.
3. Cut the bottom 1½ inches from the asparagus.
4. Heat a large skillet over medium-low heat. When hot, melt the butter in the skillet, then arrange the cod and asparagus in a single layer.
5. Cover and cook for 8 minutes.
6. Divide the rice, fish, and asparagus into four equal portions. Drizzle with the lemon juice to finish.

Per Serving
calories: 230 | fat: 8g | protein: 22g | carbs: 20g | sugars: 2g | fiber: 5g | sodium: 274mg

Tuna Casserole

Prep time: 10 minutes | Cook time: 40 minutes | Serves 4

Avocado oil cooking spray	1 cup fresh or frozen broccoli florets
1 medium yellow onion, diced	1 (10-ounce / 283-g) package zucchini noodles
2 tablespoons whole-wheat flour	2 (5-ounce / 142-g) cans chunk-light tuna, drained
2 cups low-sodium chicken broth	1 cup shredded Cheddar cheese
1 cup unsweetened almond milk	

1. Preheat the oven to 375°F (190°C).
2. Heat a medium skillet over medium heat. When hot, coat the cooking surface with cooking spray. Put the onion into the skillet and cook for 3 minutes.
3. Add the flour and stir. Cook for 2 minutes, stirring once.
4. Add the broth slowly, then the almond milk, stirring constantly.
5. Increase the heat to high. Once the mixture comes to a boil, add the broccoli and noodles. Reduce the heat to medium and cook for 5 to 7 minutes. The mixture will thicken.
6. Add the tuna and stir.
7. Transfer the mixture to an 8-by-8-inch casserole dish and top with the cheese.
8. Cover with foil and bake for 20 minutes.
9. Uncover and broil for 2 minutes.

Per Serving
calories: 269 | fat: 12g | protein: 29g | carbs: 11g | sugars: 3g | fiber: 3g | sodium: 351mg

Salsa Verde Baked Salmon

Prep time: 5 minutes | Cook time: 25 minutes | Serves 4

Nonstick cooking spray
8 ounces (227 g) tomatillos, husks removed
½ onion, quartered
1 jalapeño or serrano pepper, seeded
1 garlic clove, unpeeled
1 teaspoon extra-
virgin olive oil
½ teaspoon salt, divided
4 (4-ounce / 113-g) wild-caught salmon fillets
¼ teaspoon freshly ground black pepper
¼ cup chopped fresh cilantro
Juice of 1 lime

1. Preheat the oven to 425ºF (220ºC). Spray a baking sheet with nonstick cooking spray.
2. In a large bowl, toss the tomatillos, onion, jalapeño, garlic, olive oil, and ¼ teaspoon of salt to coat. Arrange in a single layer on the prepared baking sheet, and roast for about 10 minutes until just softened. Transfer to a dish or plate and set aside.
3. Arrange the salmon fillets skin-side down on the same baking sheet, and season with the remaining ¼ teaspoon of salt and the pepper. Bake for 12 to 15 minutes until the fish is firm and flakes easily.
4. Meanwhile, peel the roasted garlic and place it and the roasted vegetables in a blender or food processor. Add a scant ¼ cup of water to the jar, and process until smooth.
5. Add the cilantro and lime juice and process until smooth. Serve the salmon topped with the salsa verde.

Per Serving

calories: 199 | fat: 9g | protein: 23g | carbs: 6g | sugars: 3g | fiber: 2g | sodium: 295mg

Ceviche

Prep time: 10 minutes | Cook time: 0 minutes | Serves 4

½ pound (227 g) fresh skinless, white, ocean fish fillet (halibut, mahi mahi, etc.), diced
1 cup freshly squeezed lime juice, divided
2 tablespoons chopped fresh cilantro, divided
1 serrano pepper, sliced
1 garlic clove, crushed
¾ teaspoon salt, divided
½ red onion, thinly sliced
2 tomatoes, diced
1 red bell pepper, seeded and diced
1 tablespoon extra-virgin olive oil

1. In a large mixing bowl, combine the fish, ¾ cup of lime juice, 1 tablespoon of cilantro, serrano pepper, garlic, and ½ teaspoon of salt. The fish should be covered or nearly covered in lime juice. Cover the bowl and refrigerate for 4 hours.
2. Sprinkle the remaining ¼ teaspoon of salt over the onion in a small bowl, and let sit for 10 minutes. Drain and rinse well.
3. In a large bowl, combine the tomatoes, bell pepper, olive oil, remaining ¼ cup of lime juice, and onion. Let rest for at least 10 minutes, or as long as 4 hours, while the fish "cooks."
4. When the fish is ready, it will be completely white and opaque. At this time, strain the juice, reserving it in another bowl. If desired, remove the serrano pepper and garlic.
5. Add the vegetables to the fish, and stir gently. Taste, and add some of the reserved lime juice to the ceviche as desired. Serve topped with the remaining 1 tablespoon of cilantro.

Per Serving

calories: 121 | fat: 4g | protein: 12g | carbs: 11g | sugars: 5g | fiber: 2g | sodium: 405mg

Blackened Tilapia with Mango Salsa

Prep time: 15 minutes | Cook time: 10 minutes | Serves 2

Salsa:

1 cup chopped mango
2 tablespoons chopped red onion
2 tablespoons chopped fresh cilantro

2 tablespoons freshly squeezed lime juice
½ jalapeño pepper, seeded and minced
Pinch salt

Tilapia:

1 tablespoon paprika
1 teaspoon onion powder
½ teaspoon freshly ground black pepper
½ teaspoon dried thyme
½ teaspoon garlic powder

¼ teaspoon cayenne pepper
¼ teaspoon salt
½ pound (227 g) boneless tilapia fillets
2 teaspoons extra-virgin olive oil
1 lime, cut into wedges, for serving

Make the Salsa

1. In a medium bowl, toss together the mango, onion, cilantro, lime juice, jalapeño, and salt. Set aside.

Make the Tilapia

1. In a small bowl, mix the paprika, onion powder, pepper, thyme, garlic powder, cayenne, and salt. Rub the mixture on both sides of the tilapia fillets.
2. In a large skillet, heat the oil over medium heat, and cook the fish for 3 to 5 minutes on each side until the outer coating is crisp and the fish is cooked through.
3. Spoon half of the salsa over each fillet and serve with lime wedges on the side.

Per Serving

calories: 240 | fat: 8g | protein: 25g | carbs: 22g | sugars: 13g | fiber: 4g | sodium: 417mg

Baked Oysters with Vegetables

Prep time: 30 minutes | Cook time: 15 minutes | Serves 2

2 cups coarse salt, for holding the oysters
1 dozen fresh oysters, scrubbed
1 tablespoon butter
½ cup finely chopped artichoke hearts
¼ cup finely chopped scallions, both white and green parts

¼ cup finely chopped red bell pepper
1 garlic clove, minced
1 tablespoon finely chopped fresh parsley
Zest and juice of ½ lemon
Pinch salt
Freshly ground black pepper, to taste

1. Pour the coarse salt into an 8-by-8-inch baking dish and spread to evenly fill the bottom of the dish.
2. Prepare a clean surface to shuck the oysters. Using a shucking knife, insert the blade at the joint of the shell, where it hinges open and shut. Firmly apply pressure to pop the blade in, and work the knife around the shell to open. Discard the empty half of the shell. Use the knife to gently loosen the oyster, and remove any shell particles. Set the oysters in their shells on the salt, being careful not to spill the juices.
3. Preheat the oven to 425ºF (220ºC).
4. In a large skillet, melt the butter over medium heat. Add the artichoke hearts, scallions, and bell pepper, and cook for 5 to 7 minutes. Add the garlic and cook an additional minute. Remove from the heat and mix in the parsley, lemon zest and juice, and season with salt and pepper.
5. Divide the vegetable mixture evenly among the oysters and bake for 10 to 12 minutes until the vegetables are lightly browned.

Per Serving

calories: 134 | fat: 7g | protein: 6g | carbs: 11g | sugars: 7g | fiber: 2g | sodium: 281mg

Cajun Shrimp and Quinoa Casserole

Prep time: 15 minutes | Cook time: 30 minutes | Serves 6

½ cup quinoa
1 cup water
1 pound (454 g) shrimp, peeled and deveined
1½ teaspoons Cajun seasoning, divided
4 tomatoes, diced
1 tablespoon plus 2 teaspoons extra-virgin olive oil, divided
½ onion, diced
1 jalapeño pepper, seeded and minced
3 garlic cloves, minced
1 tablespoon tomato paste
¼ teaspoon freshly ground black pepper
½ cup shredded pepper jack cheese

1. In a pot, combine the quinoa and water. Bring to a boil, reduce the heat, cover, and simmer on low for 10 to 15 minutes until all the water is absorbed. Fluff with a fork.
2. Preheat the oven to 350ºF (180ºC).
3. In a large mixing bowl, toss the shrimp and ¾ teaspoon of Cajun seasoning.
4. In another bowl, toss the remaining ¾ teaspoon of Cajun seasoning with the tomatoes and 1½ teaspoons of olive oil.
5. In a large, oven-safe skillet, heat 1 tablespoon of olive oil over medium heat. Add the shrimp and cook for 2 to 3 minutes per side until they are opaque and firm. Remove from the skillet and set aside.
6. In the same skillet, heat the remaining ½ teaspoon of olive oil over medium-high heat. Add the onion, jalapeño, and garlic, and cook until the onion softens, 3 to 5 minutes.
7. Add the seasoned tomatoes, tomato paste, cooked quinoa, and pepper. Stir well to combine.
8. Return the shrimp to the skillet, placing them in a single layer on top of the quinoa. Sprinkle the cheese over the top.
9. Transfer the skillet to the oven and bake for 15 minutes. Turn the broiler on high, and broil for 2 minutes to brown the cheese. Serve.

Per Serving
calories: 255 | fat: 12g | protein: 18g | carbs: 15g | sugars: 1g | fiber: 2g | sodium: 469mg

Shrimp Burgers with Mango Salsa

Prep time: 15 minutes | Cook time: 10 minutes | Serves 4

Salsa:
1 cup diced mango
1 avocado, diced
1 scallion, both white and green parts, finely chopped
1 tablespoon chopped fresh cilantro
Juice of 1 lime
¼ teaspoon freshly ground black pepper

Burgers:
1 pound (454 g) shrimp, peeled and deveined
1 large egg
½ red bell pepper, seeded and coarsely chopped
¼ cup chopped scallions, both white and green parts
2 tablespoons fresh chopped cilantro
2 garlic cloves
¼ teaspoon freshly ground black pepper
1 tablespoon extra-virgin olive oil
4 cups mixed salad greens

Make the Salsa
1. In a small bowl, toss the mango, avocado, scallion, and cilantro. Sprinkle with the lime juice and pepper. Mix gently to combine and set aside.

Make the Burgers
1. In the bowl of a food processor, add half the shrimp and process until coarsely puréed. Add the egg, bell pepper, scallions, cilantro, and garlic, and process until uniformly chopped. Transfer to a large mixing bowl.
2. Using a sharp knife, chop the remaining half pound of shrimp into small pieces. Add to the puréed mixture and stir well to combine. Add the pepper and stir well. Form the mixture into 4 patties of equal size. Arrange on a plate, cover, and refrigerate for 30 minutes.
3. In a large skillet, heat the olive oil over medium heat. Cook the burgers for 3 minutes on each side until browned and cooked through.
4. On each of 4 plates, arrange 1 cup of salad greens, and top with a scoop of salsa and a shrimp burger.

Per Serving
calories: 229 | fat: 11g | protein: 19g | carbs: 14g | sugars: 7g | fiber: 4g | sodium: 200mg

Crab Cakes with Honeydew Melon Salsa

Prep time: 30 minutes | Cook time: 10 minutes | Serves 4

Salsa:

1 cup finely chopped honeydew melon
1 scallion, white and green parts, finely chopped
1 red bell pepper, seeded, finely chopped
1 teaspoon chopped fresh thyme
Pinch sea salt
Pinch freshly ground black pepper

Crab Cakes:

1 pound (454 g) lump crab meat, drained and picked over
¼ cup finely chopped red onion
¼ cup panko bread crumbs
1 tablespoon chopped fresh parsley
1 teaspoon lemon zest
1 egg
¼ cup whole-wheat flour
Nonstick cooking spray

Make the Salsa

1. In a small bowl, stir together the melon, scallion, bell pepper, and thyme.
2. Season the salsa with salt and pepper and set aside.

Make the Crab Cakes

1. In a medium bowl, mix together the crab, onion, bread crumbs, parsley, lemon zest, and egg until very well combined.
2. Divide the crab mixture into 8 equal portions and form them into patties about ¾-inch thick.
3. Chill the crab cakes in the refrigerator for at least 1 hour to firm them up.
4. Dredge the chilled crab cakes in the flour until lightly coated, shaking off any excess flour.
5. Place a large skillet over medium heat and lightly coat it with cooking spray.
6. Cook the crab cakes until they are golden brown, turning once, about 5 minutes per side.
7. Serve warm with the salsa.

Per Serving

calories: 232 | fat: 3g | protein: 32g | carbs: 18g | sugars: 6g | fiber: 2g | sodium: 767mg

North Carolina Fish Stew

Prep time: 20 minutes | Cook time: 20 minutes | Serves 8

½ cup seafood broth
2 large white onions, chopped
4 garlic cloves, minced
¼ cup tomato paste
1 teaspoon red pepper flakes
2 teaspoons smoked paprika
3 bay leaves
1 pound (454 g) new potatoes, halved
3 cups water
2 pounds (907 g) fish fillets, such as rockfish, striped bass, or cod, cut into ½- to 1-inch dice
8 medium eggs

1. Select the Sauté setting on an electric pressure cooker, and combine the broth, onions, garlic, tomato paste, red pepper flakes, paprika, and bay leaves. Cook for 2 minutes, or until the onions and garlic are translucent.
2. Add the potatoes and 1 cup of water.
3. Close and lock the lid, and set the pressure valve to sealing.
4. Change to the Manual setting, and cook for 3 minutes.
5. Once cooking is complete, quick-release the pressure. Carefully remove the lid.
6. Add the fish and enough of the water just to cover the fish.
7. Close and lock the lid, and set the pressure valve to sealing.
8. Select the Manual setting, and cook for 3 more minutes.
9. Once cooking is complete, quick-release the pressure. Carefully remove the lid.
10. Carefully crack the eggs one by one into the stew, keeping the yolks intact.
11. Close and lock the lid, and set the pressure valve to sealing.
12. Select the Manual setting, and cook for 1 minute.
13. Once cooking is complete, quick-release the pressure. Carefully remove the lid, discard the bay leaves, and serve in bowls.

Per Serving

calories: 218 | fat: 6g | protein: 28g | carbs: 15g | sugars: 4g | fiber: 3g | sodium: 145mg

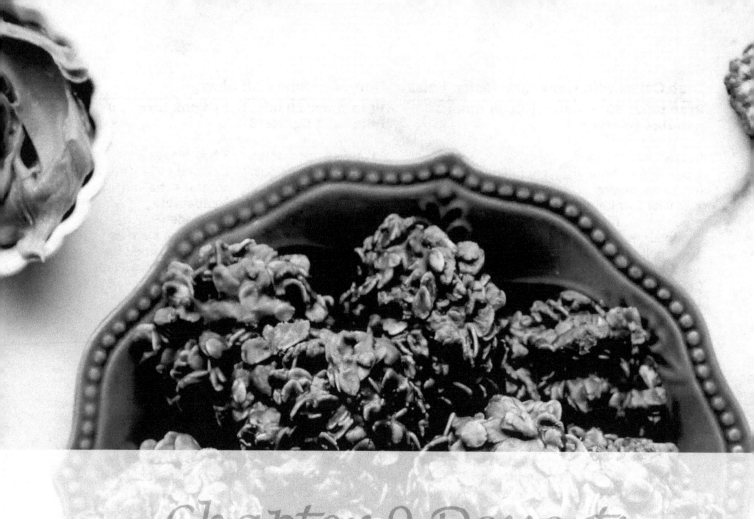
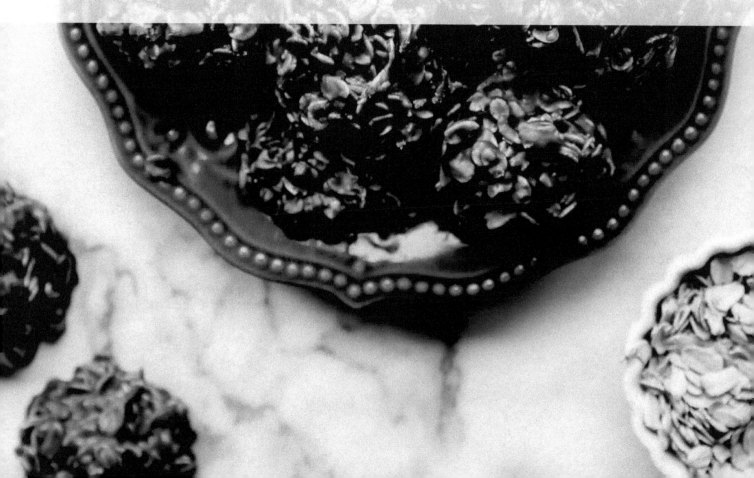

Chapter 9 Desserts

Peach and Almond Meal Fritters

Prep time: 15 minutes | Cook time: 15 minutes | Serves 7

4 ripe bananas, peeled
2 cups chopped peaches
1 medium egg
2 medium egg whites
¾ cup almond meal
¼ teaspoon almond extract

1. In a large bowl, mash the bananas and peaches together with a fork or potato masher.
2. Blend in the egg and egg whites.
3. Stir in the almond meal and almond extract.
4. Working in batches, place ¼-cup portions of the batter into the basket of an air fryer.
5. Set the air fryer to 390ºF (199ºC), close, and cook for 12 minutes.
6. Once cooking is complete, transfer the fritters to a plate. Repeat until no batter remains.

Per Serving
calories: 164 | fat: 7g | protein: 6g | carbs: 22g | sugars: 12g | fiber: 4g | sodium: 23mg

Grilled Watermelon with Avocado Mousse

Prep time: 10 minutes | Cook time: 10 minutes | Serves 8

1 small, seedless watermelon, halved and cut into 1-inch rounds
2 ripe avocados, pitted and peeled
½ cup fat-free plain yogurt
¼ teaspoon cayenne pepper

1. On a hot grill, grill the watermelon slices for 2 to 3 minutes on each side, or until you can see the grill marks.
2. To make the avocado mousse, in a blender, combine the avocados, yogurt, and cayenne and process until smooth.
3. To serve, cut each watermelon round in half. Top each with a generous dollop of avocado mousse.

Per Serving
calories: 126 | fat: 4g | protein: 3g | carbs: 24g | sugars: 17g | fiber: 3g | sodium: 14mg

No-Bake Chocolate Peanut Butter Cookies

Prep time: 10 minutes | Cook time: 0 minutes | Makes 12 cookies

¾ cup unsweetened shredded coconut
½ cup peanut butter
2 tablespoons cream cheese, at room temperature
2 tablespoons unsalted butter, melted
2 tablespoons unsweetened cocoa powder
2 tablespoons pure maple syrup
½ teaspoon vanilla extract

1. In a medium bowl, mix all of the ingredients until well combined.
2. Spoon into 12 cookies on a platter lined with parchment paper. Refrigerate to set, about 2 hours.

Per Serving (1 cookie)
calories: 143 | fat: 12g | protein: 4g | carbs: 6g | sugars: 3g | fiber: 2g | sodium: 13mg

Chocolate Almond Butter Fudge

Prep time: 10 minutes | Cook time: 0 minutes | Makes 9 pieces

2 ounces (57 g) unsweetened baking chocolate
½ cup almond butter
1 can full-fat coconut milk, refrigerated overnight, thickened cream only
1 teaspoon vanilla extract
4 (1-gram) packets stevia (or to taste)

1. Line a 9-inch square baking pan with parchment paper.
2. In a small saucepan over medium-low heat, heat the chocolate and almond butter, stirring constantly, until both are melted. Cool slightly.
3. In a medium bowl, combine the melted chocolate mixture with the cream from the coconut milk, vanilla, and stevia. Blend until smooth. Taste and adjust sweetness as desired.
4. Pour the mixture into the prepared pan, spreading with a spatula to smooth. Refrigerate for 3 hours. Cut into squares.

Per Serving (1 piece)
calories: 200 | fat: 20g | protein: 4g | carbs: 6g | sugars: 2g | fiber: 2g | sodium: 8mg

Greek Yogurt Berry Smoothie Pops

Prep time: 5 minutes | Cook time: 0 minutes | Serves 6

2 cups frozen mixed berries
½ cup unsweetened plain almond milk
1 cup plain nonfat Greek yogurt
2 tablespoons hemp seeds

1. Place all the ingredients in a blender and process until finely blended.
2. Pour into 6 clean ice pop molds and insert sticks.
3. Freeze for 3 to 4 hours until firm.

Per Serving

calories: 70 | fat: 2g | protein: 5g | carbs: 9g | sugars: 2g | fiber: 3g | sodium: 28mg

Maple Oatmeal Cookies

Prep time: 5 minutes | Cook time: 15 minutes | Serves 16

¾ cup almond flour
¾ cup old-fashioned oats
¼ cup shredded unsweetened coconut
1 teaspoon baking powder
1 teaspoon ground cinnamon
¼ teaspoon salt
¼ cup unsweetened applesauce
1 large egg
1 tablespoon pure maple syrup
2 tablespoons coconut oil, melted

1. Preheat the oven to 350ºF (180ºC).
2. In a medium mixing bowl, combine the almond flour, oats, coconut, baking powder, cinnamon, and salt, and mix well.
3. In another medium bowl, combine the applesauce, egg, maple syrup, and coconut oil, and mix. Stir the wet mixture into the dry mixture.
4. Form the dough into balls a little bigger than a tablespoon and place on a baking sheet, leaving at least 1 inch between them. Bake for 12 minutes until the cookies are just browned. Remove from the oven and let cool for 5 minutes.
5. Using a spatula, remove the cookies and cool on a rack.

Per Serving

calories: 76 | fat: 6g | protein: 2g | carbs: 5g | sugars: 1g | fiber: 1g | sodium: 57mg

Pineapple Nice Cream

Prep time: 10 minutes | Cook time: 0 minutes | Serves 6

2 cups frozen pineapple
1 cup peanut butter (no added sugar, salt,
or fat)
½ cup unsweetened almond milk

1. In a blender or food processor, combine the frozen pineapple and peanut butter and process.
2. Add the almond milk, and blend until smooth. The end result should be a smooth paste.

Per Serving

calories: 301 | fat: 22g | protein: 14g | carbs: 15g | sugars: 8g | fiber: 4g | sodium: 39mg

No-Bake Carrot Cake Bites

Prep time: 15 minutes | Cook time: 0 minutes | Serves 20

½ cup old-fashioned oats
2 medium carrots, chopped
6 dates, pitted
½ cup chopped walnuts
½ cup coconut flour
2 tablespoons hemp seeds
2 teaspoons pure maple syrup
1 teaspoon ground cinnamon
½ teaspoon ground nutmeg

1. In a blender jar, combine the oats and carrots, and process until finely ground. Transfer to a bowl.
2. Add the dates and walnuts to the blender and process until coarsely chopped. Return the oat-carrot mixture to the blender and add the coconut flour, hemp seeds, maple syrup, cinnamon, and nutmeg. Process until well mixed.
3. Using your hands, shape the dough into balls about the size of a tablespoon.
4. Store in the refrigerator in an airtight container for up to 1 week.

Per Serving

calories: 68 | fat: 3g | protein: 2g | carbs: 10g | sugars: 6g | fiber: 2g | sodium: 6mg

Spiced Orange Rice Pudding

Prep time: 5 minutes | Cook time: 35 minutes | Serves 6

2 cups short-grain brown rice
6 cups fat-free milk
1 teaspoon ground nutmeg, plus more for serving
1 teaspoon ground cinnamon, plus more for serving
¼ teaspoon orange extract
Juice of 2 oranges (about ¾ cup)
½ cup erythritol or other brown sugar replacement

1. In an electric pressure cooker, stir the rice, milk, nutmeg, cinnamon, orange extract, orange juice, and erythritol together.
2. Close and lock the lid, and set the pressure valve to sealing.
3. Select the Manual setting, and cook for 35 minutes.
4. Once cooking is complete, quick-release the pressure. Carefully remove the lid.
5. Stir well and spoon into serving dishes. Enjoy with an additional sprinkle of nutmeg and cinnamon.

Per Serving
calories: 320 | fat: 2g | protein: 13g | carbs: 61g | sugars: 15g | fiber: 2g | sodium: 130mg

Dark Chocolate Almond Butter Cups

Prep time: 15 minutes | Cook time: 0 minutes | Serves 12

½ cup natural almond butter
1 tablespoon pure maple syrup
1 cup dark chocolate chips
1 tablespoon coconut oil

1. Line a 12-cup muffin tin with cupcake liners.
2. In a medium bowl, mix the almond butter and maple syrup. If necessary, heat in the microwave to soften slightly.
3. Spoon about 2 teaspoons of the almond butter mixture into each muffin cup and press down to fill.
4. In a double boiler or the microwave, melt the chocolate chips. Stir in the coconut oil, and mix well to incorporate.
5. Drop 1 tablespoon of chocolate on top of each almond butter cup.

6. Freeze for at least 30 minutes to set. Thaw for 10 minutes before serving.

Per Serving
calories: 101 | fat: 8g | protein: 3g | carbs: 6g | sugars: 4g | fiber: 1g | sodium: 32mg

Ambrosia

Prep time: 10 minutes | Cook time: 0 minutes | Serves 8

3 oranges, peeled, sectioned, and quartered
2 (4-ounce / 113-g) cups diced peaches in water, drained
1 cup shredded, unsweetened coconut
1 (8-ounce / 227-g) container fat-free crème fraîche

1. In a large mixing bowl, combine the oranges, peaches, coconut, and crème fraîche. Gently toss until well mixed. Cover and refrigerate overnight.

Per Serving
calories: 111 | fat: 5g | protein: 2g | carbs: 12g | sugars: 8g | fiber: 3g | sodium: 7mg

Ice Cream with Strawberry Rhubarb Sauce

Prep time: 10 minutes | Cook time: 15 minutes | Serves 4

1 cup sliced strawberries
1 cup chopped rhubarb
2 tablespoons water
1 tablespoon honey
½ teaspoon cinnamon
4 (¼-cup) scoops sugar-free vanilla ice cream

1. In a medium pot, combine the strawberries, rhubarb, water, honey, and cinnamon. Bring to a simmer on medium heat, stirring. Reduce the heat to medium-low. Simmer, stirring frequently, until the rhubarb is soft, about 15 minutes. Allow to cool slightly.
2. Place 1 scoop of ice cream into each of 4 bowls. Spoon the sauce over the ice cream.

Per Serving
calories: 86 | fat: 2g | protein: 3g | carbs: 16g | sugars: 7g | fiber: 3g | sodium: 37mg

Frozen Chocolate Peanut Butter Bites

Prep time: 5 minutes | Cook time: 0 minutes | Serves 32

1 cup coconut oil, melted
¼ cup cocoa powder
¼ cup honey
¼ cup natural peanut butter

1. Pour the melted coconut oil into a medium bowl. Whisk in the cocoa powder, honey, and peanut butter.
2. Transfer the mixture to ice cube trays in portions about 1½ teaspoons each.
3. Freeze for 2 hours or until ready to serve.

Per Serving

calories: 80 | fat: 8g | protein: 1g | carbs: 3g | sugars: 2g | fiber: 0g | sodium: 20mg

Flourless Orange Bundt Cake

Prep time: 15 minutes | Cook time: 30 minutes | Serves 24

Unsalted non-hydrogenated plant-based butter, for greasing the pan
1½ cups gluten-free baking flour, plus more for dusting
1½ cups almond flour
½ teaspoon baking soda
½ teaspoon baking powder
9 medium eggs, at room temperature
1 cup coconut sugar
Zest of 3 oranges
Juice of 1 orange
1 cup extra-virgin olive oil

1. Preheat the oven to 325ºF (163ºC).
2. Grease two bundt pans with butter and dust with the baking flour.
3. In a medium bowl, whisk the baking flour, almond flour, baking soda, and baking powder together.
4. In a large bowl, whip the eggs with the coconut sugar until they double in size.
5. Add the orange zest and orange juice.
6. Add the dry ingredients to the wet ingredients, stirring to combine.
7. Add the olive oil, a little at a time, until incorporated.
8. Divide the batter between the two prepared bundt pans.
9. Transfer the bundt pans to the oven, and bake for 30 minutes, or until browned and a toothpick inserted into the center comes out clean.
10. Remove the bundt pans from the oven, and let cool for 15 minutes.
11. Invert the bundt pans onto plates, and gently tap the cakes out of the pan.

Per Serving

calories: 179 | fat: 12g | protein: 4g | carbs: 15g | sugars: 8g | fiber: 1g | sodium: 52mg

Air Fryer Apples

Prep time: 5 minutes | Cook time: 15 minutes | Serves 6 to 8

4 Pink Lady apples, quartered
¼ cup erythritol or
other brown sugar replacement

1. In a small mixing bowl, toss the apples in the erythritol. Working in batches, place in the basket of an air fryer.
2. Set the air fryer to 390ºF (199ºC), close, and cook for 15 minutes.
3. Once cooking is complete, transfer the apples to a plate. Repeat until no apples remain.

Per Serving

calories: 47 | fat: 0g | protein: 0g | carbs: 11g | sugars: 8g | fiber: 2g | sodium: 0mg

Coffee and Cream Pops

Prep time: 10 minutes | Cook time: 5 minutes | Serves 4

2 teaspoons espresso powder (or to taste)
2 cups canned coconut milk
½ teaspoon vanilla
extract
½ teaspoon cinnamon
3 (1-gram) packets stevia

1. In a medium saucepan over medium-low heat, heat all of the ingredients, stirring constantly, until the espresso powder is completely dissolved, about 5 minutes.
2. Pour the mixture into 4 ice pop molds. Freeze for 6 hours before serving.

Per Serving

calories: 225 | fat: 24g | protein: 2g | carbs: 7g | sugars: 1g | fiber: 3g | sodium: 15mg

Creamy Strawberry Crepes

Prep time: 10 minutes | Cook time: 10 minutes | Serves 4

½ cup old-fashioned oats
1 cup unsweetened plain almond milk
1 egg
3 teaspoons honey, divided
Nonstick cooking
spray
2 ounces (57 g) low-fat cream cheese
¼ cup low-fat cottage cheese
2 cups sliced strawberries

1. In a blender jar, process the oats until they resemble flour. Add the almond milk, egg, and 1½ teaspoons honey, and process until smooth.
2. Heat a large skillet over medium heat. Spray with nonstick cooking spray to coat.
3. Add ¼ cup of oat batter to the pan and quickly swirl around to coat the bottom of the pan and let cook for 2 to 3 minutes. When the edges begin to turn brown, flip the crepe with a spatula and cook until lightly browned and firm, about 1 minute. Transfer to a plate. Continue with the remaining batter, spraying the skillet with nonstick cooking spray before adding more batter. Set the cooked crepes aside, loosely covered with aluminum foil, while you make the filling.
4. Clean the blender jar, then combine the cream cheese, cottage cheese, and remaining 1½ teaspoons honey, and process until smooth.
5. Fill each crepe with 2 tablespoons of the cream cheese mixture, topped with ¼ cup of strawberries. Serve.

Per Serving
calories: 149 | fat: 6g | protein: 6g | carbs: 20g | sugars: 10g | fiber: 3g | sodium: 177mg

Goat Cheese-Stuffed Pears

Prep time: 6 minutes | Cook time: 2 minutes | Serves 4

2 ounces (57 g) goat cheese, at room temperature
2 teaspoons pure maple syrup
2 ripe, firm pears,
halved lengthwise and cored
2 tablespoons chopped pistachios, toasted

1. Pour 1 cup of water into the electric pressure cooker and insert a wire rack or trivet.
2. In a small bowl, combine the goat cheese and maple syrup.
3. Spoon the goat cheese mixture into the cored pear halves. Place the pears on the rack inside the pot, cut-side up.
4. Close and lock the lid of the pressure cooker. Set the valve to sealing.
5. Cook on high pressure for 2 minutes.
6. When the cooking is complete, hit Cancel and quick release the pressure.
7. Once the pin drops, unlock and remove the lid.
8. Using tongs, carefully transfer the pears to serving plates.
9. Sprinkle with pistachios and serve immediately.

Per Serving (½ pear)
calories: 120 | fat: 5g | protein: 4g | carbs: 17g | sugars: 11g | fiber: 3g | sodium: 54mg

Spiced Pear Applesauce

Prep time: 15 minutes | Cook time: 5 minutes | Makes 3½ cups

2 pounds (907 g) apples, peeled, cored, and sliced
1 pound (454 g) pears, peeled, cored, and sliced
2 teaspoons apple pie spice or cinnamon
Pinch kosher salt
Juice of ½ small lemon

1. In the electric pressure cooker, combine the apples, pears, apple pie spice, salt, lemon juice, and ¼ cup of water.
2. Close and lock the lid of the pressure cooker. Set the valve to sealing.
3. Cook on high pressure for 5 minutes.
4. When the cooking is complete, hit Cancel and let the pressure release naturally.
5. Once the pin drops, unlock and remove the lid.
6. Mash the apples and pears with a potato masher to the consistency you like.
7. Serve warm, or cool to room temperature and refrigerate.

Per Serving (½ cup)
calories: 108 | fat: 1g | protein: 1g | carbs: 29g | sugars: 20g | fiber: 6g | sodium: 15mg

Golden Potato Cakes

Prep time: 10 minutes | Cook time: 25 minutes | Serves 4

½ pound (227 g) russet potatoes, peeled, shredded, rinsed, and patted dry
¼ sweet onion, chopped
1 teaspoon extra-virgin olive oil

1 teaspoon chopped fresh thyme
Sea salt and freshly ground black pepper, to taste
Nonstick cooking spray
1 cup unsweetened applesauce

1. Place the potatoes, onion, oil, and thyme in a large bowl and stir to mix well.
2. Season the potato mixture generously with salt and pepper.
3. Place a large skillet over medium heat and lightly coat it with cooking spray.
4. Scoop about ¼ cup of potato mixture per cake into the skillet and press down with a spatula, about 4 cakes per batch.
5. Cook until the bottoms are golden brown and firm, about 5 to 7 minutes, then flip the cake over. Cook the other side until it is golden brown and the cake is completely cooked through, about 5 minutes more.
6. Remove the cakes to a plate and repeat with the remaining mixture.
7. Serve with the applesauce.

Per Serving
calories: 106 | fat: 3g | protein: 1g | carbs: 18g | sugars: 7g | fiber: 2g | sodium: 6mg

Grilled Peach and Coconut Yogurt Bowls

Prep time: 5 minutes | Cook time: 10 minutes | Serves 4

2 peaches, halved and pitted
½ cup plain nonfat Greek yogurt
1 teaspoon pure vanilla extract

¼ cup unsweetened dried coconut flakes
2 tablespoons unsalted pistachios, shelled and broken into pieces

1. Preheat the broiler to high. Arrange the rack in the closest position to the broiler.
2. In a shallow pan, arrange the peach halves, cut-side up. Broil for 6 to 8 minutes until browned, tender, and hot.

3. In a small bowl, mix the yogurt and vanilla.
4. Spoon the yogurt into the cavity of each peach half.
5. Sprinkle 1 tablespoon of coconut flakes and 1½ teaspoons of pistachios over each peach half. Serve warm.

Per Serving
calories: 102 | fat: 5g | protein: 5g | carbs: 11g | sugars: 8g | fiber: 2g | sodium: 12mg

Cinnamon Spiced Baked Apples

Prep time: 10 minutes | Cook time: 15 minutes | Serves 4

2 apples, peeled, cored, and chopped
2 tablespoons pure maple syrup
½ teaspoon cinnamon

½ teaspoon ground ginger
¼ cup chopped pecans

1. Preheat the oven to 350ºF (180ºC).
2. In a bowl, mix the apples, syrup, cinnamon, and ginger. Pour the mixture into a 9-inch square baking dish. Sprinkle the pecans over the top.
3. Bake until the apples are tender, about 15 minutes.

Per Serving
calories: 122 | fat: 5g | protein: 1g | carbs: 21g | sugars: 13g | fiber: 3g | sodium: 2mg

Blackberry Yogurt Ice Pops

Prep time: 10 minutes | Cook time: 0 minutes | Serves 4

12 ounces (340 g) plain Greek yogurt
1 cup blackberries
Pinch nutmeg

¼ cup milk
2 (1-gram) packets stevia

1. In a blender, combine all of the ingredients. Blend until smooth.
2. Pour the mixture into 4 ice pop molds. Freeze for 6 hours before serving.

Per Serving
calories: 75 | fat: 6g | protein: 9g | carbs: 9g | sugars: 5g | fiber: 2g | sodium: 7mg

Pumpkin Cheesecake Smoothie

Prep time: 10 minutes | Cook time: 0 minutes | Serves 1

2 tablespoons cream cheese, at room temperature
½ cup canned pumpkin purée (not pumpkin pie mix)
1 cup almond milk
1 teaspoon pumpkin pie spice
½ cup crushed ice

1. In a blender, combine all of the ingredients. Blend until smooth.

Per Serving
calories: 186 | fat: 14g | protein: 5g | carbs: 14g | sugars: 10g | fiber: 5g | sodium: 105mg

Broiled Pineapple

Prep time: 5 minutes | Cook time: 5 minutes | Serves 4

4 large slices fresh pineapple
2 tablespoons canned coconut milk
2 tablespoons unsweetened shredded coconut
¼ teaspoon sea salt

1. Preheat the oven broiler on high.
2. On a rimmed baking sheet, arrange the pineapple in a single layer. Brush lightly with the coconut milk and sprinkle with the coconut.
3. Broil until the pineapple begins to brown, 3 to 5 minutes.
4. Sprinkle with the sea salt.

Per Serving
calories: 78 | fat: 4g | protein: 1g | carbs: 13g | sugars: 16g | fiber: 2g | sodium: 148mg

Avocado Chocolate Mousse

Prep time: 5 minutes | Cook time: 0 minutes | Serves 4

2 avocados, mashed
¼ cup canned coconut milk
2 tablespoons unsweetened cocoa powder
2 tablespoons pure maple syrup
½ teaspoon espresso powder
½ teaspoon vanilla extract

1. In a blender, combine all of the ingredients. Blend until smooth.

2. Pour the mixture into 4 small bowls and serve.

Per Serving
calories: 203 | fat: 17g | protein: 2g | carbs: 15g | sugars: 6g | fiber: 6g | sodium: 11mg

Chocolate Chip Banana Cake

Prep time: 15 minutes | Cook time: 25 minutes | Serves 8

Nonstick cooking spray
3 ripe bananas
½ cup buttermilk
3 tablespoons honey
1 teaspoon vanilla extract
2 large eggs, lightly beaten
3 tablespoons extra-virgin olive oil
1½ cups whole wheat pastry flour
⅛ teaspoon ground nutmeg
1 teaspoon ground cinnamon
¼ teaspoon salt
1 teaspoon baking soda
⅓ cup dark chocolate chips

1. Spray a 7-inch Bundt pan with nonstick cooking spray.
2. In a large bowl, mash the bananas. Add the buttermilk, honey, vanilla, eggs, and olive oil, and mix well.
3. In a medium bowl, whisk together the flour, nutmeg, cinnamon, salt, and baking soda.
4. Add the flour mixture to the banana mixture and mix well. Stir in the chocolate chips. Pour the batter into the prepared Bundt pan. Cover the pan with foil.
5. Pour 1 cup of water into the electric pressure cooker. Place the pan on the wire rack and lower it into the pressure cooker.
6. Close and lock the lid of the pressure cooker. Set the valve to sealing.
7. Cook on high pressure for 25 minutes.
8. When the cooking is complete, hit Cancel and quick release the pressure.
9. Once the pin drops, unlock and remove the lid.
10. Carefully transfer the pan to a cooling rack, uncover, and let it cool for 10 minutes.
11. Invert the cake onto the rack and let it cool for about an hour.
12. Slice and serve the cake.

Per Serving (1 slice)
calories: 261 | fat: 11g | protein: 6g | carbs: 39g | sugars: 16g | fiber: 4g | sodium: 239mg

Apple Crunch

Prep time: 13 minutes | Cook time: 2 minutes | Serves 4

3 apples, peeled, cored, and sliced (about 1½ pounds / 680 g)
1 teaspoon pure maple syrup
1 teaspoon apple pie spice or ground cinnamon
¼ cup unsweetened apple juice, apple cider, or water
¼ cup low-sugar granola

1. In the electric pressure cooker, combine the apples, maple syrup, apple pie spice, and apple juice.
2. Close and lock the lid of the pressure cooker. Set the valve to sealing.
3. Cook on high pressure for 2 minutes.
4. When the cooking is complete, hit Cancel and quick release the pressure.
5. Once the pin drops, unlock and remove the lid.
6. Spoon the apples into 4 serving bowls and sprinkle each with 1 tablespoon of granola.

Per Serving
calories: 103 | fat: 1g | protein: 1g | carbs: 26g | sugars: 18g | fiber: 4g | sodium: 13mg

Chai Pear-Fig Compote

Prep time: 20 minutes | Cook time: 3 minutes | Serves 4

1 vanilla chai tea bag
1 (3-inch) cinnamon stick
1 strip lemon peel (about 2-by-½ inches)
1½ pounds (680 g) pears, peeled and chopped (about 3 cups)
½ cup chopped dried figs
2 tablespoons raisins

1. Pour 1 cup of water into the electric pressure cooker and hit Sauté/More. When the water comes to a boil, add the tea bag and cinnamon stick. Hit Cancel. Let the tea steep for 5 minutes, then remove and discard the tea bag.
2. Add the lemon peel, pears, figs, and raisins to the pot.
3. Close and lock the lid of the pressure cooker. Set the valve to sealing.
4. Cook on high pressure for 3 minutes.

5. When the cooking is complete, hit Cancel and quick release the pressure.
6. Once the pin drops, unlock and remove the lid.
7. Remove the lemon peel and cinnamon stick. Serve warm or cool to room temperature and refrigerate.

Per Serving
calories: 167 | fat: 1g | protein: 2g | carbs: 44g | sugars: 29g | fiber: 9g | sodium: 4mg

Bran Apple Muffins

Prep time: 10 minutes | Cook time: 20 minutes | Makes 18 muffins

2 cups whole-wheat flour
1 cup wheat bran
1/3 cup granulated sweetener
1 tablespoon baking powder
2 teaspoons ground cinnamon
½ teaspoon ground ginger
¼ teaspoon ground nutmeg
Pinch sea salt
2 eggs
1½ cups skim milk, at room temperature
½ cup melted coconut oil
2 teaspoons pure vanilla extract
2 apples, peeled, cored, and diced

1. Preheat the oven to 350ºF (180ºC).
2. Line 18 muffin cups with paper liners and set the tray aside.
3. In a large bowl, stir together the flour, bran, sweetener, baking powder, cinnamon, ginger, nutmeg, and salt.
4. In a small bowl, whisk the eggs, milk, coconut oil, and vanilla until blended.
5. Add the wet ingredients to the dry ingredients, stirring until just blended.
6. Stir in the apples and spoon equal amounts of batter into each muffin cup.
7. Bake the muffins until a toothpick inserted in the center of a muffin comes out clean, about 20 minutes.
8. Cool the muffins completely and serve.
9. Store leftover muffins in a sealed container in the refrigerator for up to 3 days or in the freezer for up to 1 month.

Per Serving
calories: 141 | fat: 7g | protein: 4g | carbs: 19g | sugars: g6 | fiber: 3g | sodium: 20mg

Cottage Cheese Almond Pancakes

Prep time: 10 minutes | Cook time: 20 minutes | Serves 4

2 cups low-fat cottage cheese
4 egg whites
2 eggs
1 tablespoon pure

vanilla extract
1½ cups almond flour
Nonstick cooking spray

1. Place the cottage cheese, egg whites, eggs, and vanilla in a blender and pulse to combine.
2. Add the almond flour to the blender and blend until smooth.
3. Place a large nonstick skillet over medium heat and lightly coat it with cooking spray.
4. Spoon ¼ cup of batter per pancake, 4 at a time, into the skillet. Cook the pancakes until the bottoms are firm and golden, about 4 minutes.
5. Flip the pancakes over and cook the other side until they are cooked through, about 3 minutes.
6. Remove the pancakes to a plate and repeat with the remaining batter.
7. Serve with fresh fruit.

Per Serving
calories: 344 | fat: 22g | protein: 29g | carbs: 11g | sugars: 5g | fiber: 4g | sodium: 559mg

Greek Yogurt Cinnamon Pancakes

Prep time: 5 minutes | Cook time: 20 minutes | Serves 4

1 cup 2 percent plain Greek yogurt
3 eggs
1½ teaspoons pure vanilla extract
1 cup rolled oats
1 tablespoon granulated sweetener

1 teaspoon baking powder
1 teaspoon ground cinnamon
Pinch ground cloves
Nonstick cooking spray

1. Place the yogurt, eggs, and vanilla in a blender and pulse to combine.
2. Add the oats, sweetener, baking powder, cinnamon, and cloves to the blender and blend until the batter is smooth.
3. Place a large nonstick skillet over medium heat and lightly coat it with cooking spray.
4. Spoon ¼ cup of batter per pancake, 4 at a time, into the skillet. Cook the pancakes until the bottoms are firm and golden, about 4 minutes.
5. Flip the pancakes over and cook the other side until they are cooked through, about 3 minutes.
6. Remove the pancakes to a plate and repeat with the remaining batter.
7. Serve with fresh fruit.

Per Serving
calories: 243 | fat: 8g | protein: 13g | carbs: 28g | sugars: 3g | fiber: 4g | sodium: 81mg

Swirled Cream Cheese Brownies

Prep time: 10 minutes | Cook time: 20 minutes | Serves 12

2 eggs
¼ cup unsweetened applesauce
¼ cup coconut oil, melted
3 tablespoons pure maple syrup, divided
¼ cup unsweetened

cocoa powder
¼ cup coconut flour
¼ teaspoon salt
1 teaspoon baking powder
2 tablespoons low-fat cream cheese

1. Preheat the oven to 350ºF (180ºC). Grease an 8-by-8-inch baking dish.
2. In a large mixing bowl, beat the eggs with the applesauce, coconut oil, and 2 tablespoons of maple syrup.
3. Stir in the cocoa powder and coconut flour, and mix well. Sprinkle the salt and baking powder evenly over the surface and mix well to incorporate. Transfer the mixture to the prepared baking dish.
4. In a small, microwave-safe bowl, microwave the cream cheese for 10 to 20 seconds until softened. Add the remaining 1 tablespoon of maple syrup and mix to combine.
5. Drop the cream cheese onto the batter, and use a toothpick or chopstick to swirl it on the surface. Bake for 20 minutes, until a toothpick inserted in the center comes out clean. Cool and cut into 12 squares.
6. Store refrigerated in a covered container for up to 5 days.

Per Serving
calories: 84 | fat: 6g | protein: 2g | carbs: 6g | sugars: 4g | fiber: 2g | sodium: 93mg

Tapioca Berry Parfaits

Prep time: 10 minutes | Cook time: 6 minutes | Serves 4

2 cups unsweetened almond milk
½ cup small pearl tapioca, rinsed and still wet
1 teaspoon almond extract
1 tablespoon pure maple syrup
2 cups berries
¼ cup slivered almonds

1. Pour the almond milk into the electric pressure cooker. Stir in the tapioca and almond extract.
2. Close and lock the lid of the pressure cooker. Set the valve to sealing.
3. Cook on High pressure for 6 minutes.
4. When the cooking is complete, hit Cancel. Allow the pressure to release naturally for 10 minutes, then quick release any remaining pressure.
5. Once the pin drops, unlock and remove the lid. Remove the pot to a cooling rack.
6. Stir in the maple syrup and let the mixture cool for about an hour.
7. In small glasses, create several layers of tapioca, berries, and almonds. Refrigerate for 1 hour.
8. Serve chilled.

Per Serving (6 tablespoons tapioca, ½ cup berries, and 1 tablespoon almonds)
calories: 174 | fat: 5g | protein: 3g | carbs: 32g | sugars: 11g | fiber: 3g | sodium: 77mg

Pumpkin Apple Waffles

Prep time: 10 minutes | Cook time: 20 minutes | Serves 6

2¼ cups whole-wheat pastry flour
2 tablespoons granulated sweetener
1 tablespoon baking powder
1 teaspoon ground cinnamon
1 teaspoon ground nutmeg
4 eggs
1¼ cups pure pumpkin purée
1 apple, peeled, cored, and finely chopped
Melted coconut oil, for cooking

1. In a large bowl, stir together the flour, sweetener, baking powder, cinnamon, and nutmeg.
2. In a small bowl, whisk together the eggs and pumpkin.
3. Add the wet ingredients to the dry and whisk until smooth.
4. Stir the apple into the batter.
5. Cook the waffles according to the waffle maker manufacturer's directions, brushing your waffle iron with melted coconut oil, until all the batter is gone.
6. Serve.

Per Serving
calories: 231 | fat: 4g | protein: 11g | carbs: 40g | sugars: 5g | fiber: 7g | sodium: 51mg

Buckwheat Crêpes with Fruit and Yogurt

Prep time: 20 minutes | Cook time: 20 minutes | Serves 5

1½ cups skim milk
3 eggs
1 teaspoon extra-virgin olive oil, plus more for the skillet
1 cup buckwheat flour
½ cup whole-wheat flour
½ cup 2 percent plain Greek yogurt
1 cup sliced strawberries
1 cup blueberries

1. In a large bowl, whisk together the milk, eggs, and 1 teaspoon of oil until well combined.
2. Into a medium bowl, sift together the buckwheat and whole-wheat flours. Add the dry ingredients to the wet ingredients and whisk until well combined and very smooth.
3. Allow the batter to rest for at least 2 hours before cooking.
4. Place a large skillet or crêpe pan over medium-high heat and lightly coat the bottom with oil.
5. Pour about ¼ cup of batter into the skillet. Swirl the pan until the batter completely coats the bottom.
6. Cook the crêpe for about 1 minute, then flip it over. Cook the other side of the crêpe for another minute, until lightly browned. Transfer the cooked crêpe to a plate and cover with a clean dish towel to keep warm.
7. Repeat until the batter is used up; you should have about 10 crêpes.
8. Spoon 1 tablespoon of yogurt onto each crêpe and place two crêpes on each plate.
9. Top with berries and serve.

Per Serving (2 crêpes)
calories: 329 | fat: 7g | protein: 16g | carbs: 54g | sugars: 11g | fiber: 8g | sodium: 102mg

Banana Pudding

Prep time: 30 minutes | Cook time: 20 minutes | Serves 10

Pudding:

¾ cup erythritol or other sugar replacement
5 teaspoons almond flour
¼ teaspoon salt
2½ cups fat-free milk
6 tablespoons prepared egg replacement
½ teaspoon vanilla extract
2 (8-ounce / 227-g) containers sugar-free spelt hazelnut biscuits, crushed
5 medium bananas, sliced

Meringue:

5 medium egg whites (1 cup)
¼ cup erythritol or other sugar replacement
½ teaspoon vanilla extract

Make the Pudding

1. In a saucepan, whisk the erythritol, almond flour, salt, and milk together. Cook over medium heat until the sugar is dissolved.
2. Whisk in the egg replacement and cook for about 10 minutes, or until thickened.
3. Remove from the heat and stir in the vanilla.
4. Spread the thickened pudding onto the bottom of a 3 × 6-inch casserole dish.
5. Arrange a layer of crushed biscuits on top of the pudding.
6. Place a layer of sliced bananas on top of the biscuits.

Make the Meringue

1. Preheat the oven to 350ºF (180ºC).
2. In a medium bowl, beat the egg whites for about 5 minutes, or until stiff.
3. Add the erythritol and vanilla while continuing to beat for about 3 more minutes.
4. Spread the meringue on top of the banana pudding.
5. Transfer the casserole dish to the oven, and bake for 7 to 10 minutes, or until the top is lightly browned.

Per Serving

calories: 323 | fat: 14g | protein: 12g | carbs: 42g | sugars: 11g | fiber: 3g | sodium: 148mg

Chipotle Black Bean Brownies

Prep time: 15 minutes | Cook time: 30 minutes | Serves 8

Nonstick cooking spray
½ cup dark chocolate chips, divided
¾ cup cooked calypso beans or black beans
½ cup extra-virgin olive oil
2 large eggs
¼ cup unsweetened dark chocolate cocoa powder
¹⁄₃ cup honey
1 teaspoon vanilla extract
¹⁄₃ cup white wheat flour
½ teaspoon chipotle chili powder
½ teaspoon ground cinnamon
½ teaspoon baking powder
½ teaspoon kosher salt

1. Spray a 7-inch Bundt pan with nonstick cooking spray.
2. Place half of the chocolate chips in a small bowl and microwave them for 30 seconds. Stir and repeat, if necessary, until the chips have completely melted.
3. In a food processor, blend the beans and oil together. Add the melted chocolate chips, eggs, cocoa powder, honey, and vanilla. Blend until the mixture is smooth.
4. In a large bowl, whisk together the flour, chili powder, cinnamon, baking powder, and salt. Pour the bean mixture from the food processor into the bowl and stir with a wooden spoon until well combined. Stir in the remaining chocolate chips.
5. Pour the batter into the prepared Bundt pan. Cover loosely with foil.
6. Pour 1 cup of water into the electric pressure cooker.
7. Place the Bundt pan onto the wire rack and lower it into the pressure cooker.
8. Close and lock the lid of the pressure cooker. Set the valve to sealing.
9. Cook on high pressure for 30 minutes.
10. When the cooking is complete, hit Cancel and quick release the pressure.
11. Once the pin drops, unlock and remove the lid.
12. Carefully transfer the pan to a cooling rack for about 10 minutes, then invert the cake onto the rack and let it cool completely.
13. Cut into slices and serve.

Per Serving (1 slice)

calories: 296 | fat: 20g | protein: 5g | carbs: 29g | sugars: 16g | fiber: 4g | sodium: 224mg

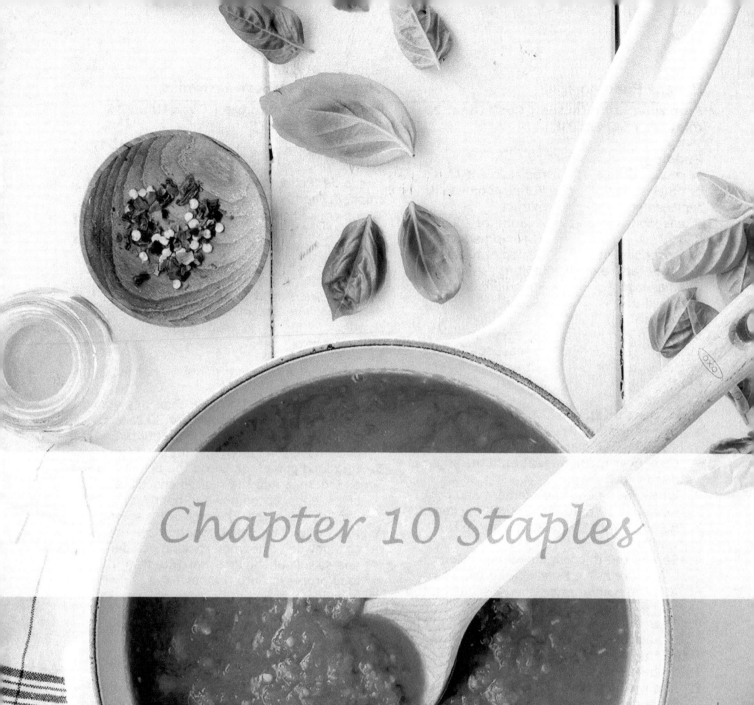

Chapter 10 Staples

Tomato Ketchup

Prep time: 10 minutes | Cook time: 0 minutes | Serves 32

1 (28-ounce / 794-g) can whole tomatoes, drained
2 (6-ounce / 170-g) cans tomato paste
1 tablespoon olive oil
2 garlic cloves, peeled
⅓ cup apple cider
vinegar
1 tablespoon dried minced onion
½ teaspoon ground cloves
1 teaspoon salt
¼ cup honey

1. In a blender jar, combine the tomatoes, tomato paste, olive oil, garlic, vinegar, onion, cloves, salt, and honey. Process until smooth. Taste and adjust the spices and seasonings as needed.
2. Transfer to airtight storage jars, cover tightly, and refrigerate for up to 3 weeks.

Per Serving

calories: 29 | fat: 1g | protein: 1g | carbs: 6g | sugars: 5g | fiber: 1g | sodium: 104mg

Beet Yogurt Dip

Prep time: 10 minutes | Cook time: 45 to 60 minutes | Serves 6

½ pound (227 g) red beets
½ cup plain nonfat Greek yogurt
1 tablespoon extra-virgin olive oil
1 tablespoon freshly
squeezed lemon juice
1 garlic clove, peeled
1 teaspoon minced fresh thyme
½ teaspoon onion powder
¼ teaspoon salt

1. Preheat the oven to 375ºF (190ºC).
2. Wrap the beets in aluminum foil and bake for 45 to 60 minutes until the beets are tender when pierced with a fork. Set aside and let cool for at least 10 minutes. Using your hands, remove the skins and transfer the beets to a blender.
3. To the blender jar, add the yogurt, olive oil, lemon juice, garlic, thyme, onion powder, and salt. Process until smooth. Chill for 1 hour before serving.

Per Serving

calories: 49 | fat: 2g | protein: 3g | carbs: 5g | sugars: 2g | fiber: 1g | sodium: 121mg

Ranch Dressing

Prep time: 10 minutes | Cook time: 0 minutes | Serves 8 to 10

8 ounces (227 g) fat-free plain Greek yogurt
¼ cup low-fat buttermilk
1 tablespoon garlic powder
1 tablespoon dried dill
1 tablespoon dried chives
1 tablespoon onion powder
1 tablespoon dried parsley
Pinch freshly ground black pepper

1. In a shallow, medium bowl, combine the Greek yogurt and buttermilk.
2. Stir in the garlic powder, dill, chives, onion powder, parsley, and pepper and mix well.
3. Serve with animal protein or vegetable of your choice, or place in an airtight container.

Per Serving

calories: 29 | fat: 0g | protein: 3g | carbs: 3g | sugars: 2g | fiber: 0g | sodium: 23mg

Ranch Vegetable Dip and Dressing

Prep time: 10 minutes | Cook time: 0 minutes | Serves 8

2 cups frozen cauliflower, thawed
½ cup unsweetened plain almond milk
2 tablespoons extra-virgin olive oil
2 tablespoons apple cider vinegar
1 garlic clove, peeled
2 teaspoons finely chopped scallions, both white and green
parts
2 teaspoons finely chopped fresh parsley
1 teaspoon finely chopped fresh dill
½ teaspoon Dijon mustard
½ teaspoon onion powder
½ teaspoon salt
¼ teaspoon freshly ground black pepper

1. In a blender jar, combine the cauliflower, almond milk, oil, vinegar, garlic, scallions, parsley, dill, mustard, onion powder, salt, and pepper. Process until very smooth.
2. Serve immediately, or transfer to a jar, cover tightly with a lid, and store in the refrigerator for up to 3 days.

Per Serving

calories: 42 | fat: 4g | protein: 1g | carbs: 2g | sugars: 1g | fiber: 1g | sodium: 149mg

Creole Seasoning

Prep time: 10 minutes | Cook time: 0 minutes | Makes ¾ cup

2 tablespoons garlic powder
2 tablespoons dried basil
1 tablespoon sweet paprika
1 tablespoon smoked paprika
1 tablespoon freshly ground black pepper

1 tablespoon onion powder
1 tablespoon cayenne pepper
1 tablespoon dried thyme
1 tablespoon dried oregano
1 teaspoon ground red sweet pepper

1. In an airtight container, combine the garlic powder, basil, sweet paprika, smoked paprika, black pepper, onion powder, cayenne, thyme, oregano, and sweet pepper.

Per Serving
calories: 13 | fat: 0g | protein: 1g | carbs: 3g | sugars: 1g | fiber: 1g | sodium: 2mg

5-Minute Pesto

Prep time: 5 minutes | Cook time: 0 minutes | Makes 1 cup

3 garlic cloves, peeled
2 cups packed fresh basil leaves
½ cup freshly grated Parmesan cheese
⅓ cup pine nuts

½ cup extra-virgin olive oil
Kosher salt and freshly ground black pepper, to taste

1. With the motor running, drop the garlic cloves through the feed tube of a food processor fitted with the steel blade. Stop the motor, then add the basil, Parmesan, and pine nuts. Pulse a few times until the pine nuts are finely minced.
2. With the motor running, add the olive oil in a steady stream and process until the pesto is completely puréed. Season with salt and pepper.
3. Store, covered, in the refrigerator for up to 2 weeks.

Per Serving (1 tablespoon)
calories: 94 | fat: 10g | protein: 2g | carbs: 1g | sugars: 0g | fiber: 0g | sodium: 71mg

Guacamole

Prep time: 10 minutes | Cook time: 0 minutes | Serves 6

2 large avocados
1 small, firm tomato, finely diced
¼ white onion, finely diced
¼ cup finely chopped

fresh cilantro
2 tablespoons freshly squeezed lime juice
¼ teaspoon salt
Freshly ground black pepper, to taste

1. Cut the avocados in half, remove the seeds, and scoop out the flesh into a medium bowl.
2. Using a fork, mash the avocado flesh. Mix in the tomato, onion, cilantro, lime juice, and salt. Season with black pepper.
3. Serve immediately.

Per Serving
calories: 82 | fat: 7g | protein: 1g | carbs: 6g | sugars: 1g | fiber: 3g | sodium: 84mg

Roasted Tomatillo Salsa

Prep time: 5 minutes | Cook time: 1 hour | Makes 1 cup

1 pound (454 g) tomatillos (about 6 large), papery husks removed, rinsed
½ large onion, quartered
3 serrano chiles, halved lengthwise,

seeded
1 tablespoon extra-virgin olive oil
1 teaspoon kosher salt
1 cup (loosely packed) fresh cilantro leaves

1. Preheat the oven to 375ºF (190ºC).
2. In an 8-inch square baking dish, combine the tomatillos, onion, chiles, oil, and salt. Roast for 1 hour or until the vegetables are very soft. Remove from the oven and let cool slightly.
3. Transfer everything from the baking dish to a food processor, and add the cilantro. Purée until almost smooth. Pour the salsa into a glass jar and store, covered, in the refrigerator for up to 1 week.

Per Serving (2 tablespoons)
calories: 33 | fat: 2g | protein: 1g | carbs: 4g | sugars: 2g | fiber: 1g | sodium: 187mg

Tzatziki

Prep time: 10 minutes | Cook time: 0 minutes | Serves 6

1 medium cucumber, peeled and grated
¼ teaspoon salt
1 cup plain nonfat Greek yogurt
2 garlic cloves, minced
1 tablespoon freshly squeezed lemon juice
1 tablespoon extra-virgin olive oil
¼ teaspoon freshly ground black pepper

1. In a colander, sprinkle the cucumber with the salt. Set aside.
2. In a medium bowl, combine the yogurt, garlic, lemon juice, olive oil, and pepper.
3. Using your hands, squeeze as much water from the grated cucumber as possible. Transfer the cucumber to the yogurt mixture and stir well. Cover and refrigerate for 2 hours, if desired, to let the flavors merge.
4. Store in the refrigerator in an airtight container for up to 5 to 7 days.

Per Serving

calories: 48 | fat: 3g | protein: 4g | carbs: 3g | sugars: 2g | fiber: 0g | sodium: 104mg

Not Old Bay Seasoning

Prep time: 10 minutes | Cook time: 0 minutes | Makes about ½ cup

3 tablespoons sweet paprika
2 tablespoons celery seeds
1 tablespoon mustard seeds
2 teaspoons freshly ground black pepper
1½ teaspoons cayenne pepper
1 teaspoon red pepper flakes
½ teaspoon ground nutmeg
½ teaspoon ground cinnamon
½ teaspoon ground ginger
¼ teaspoon ground cloves

1. In an airtight container, combine the paprika, celery seeds, mustard seeds, black pepper, cayenne, red pepper flakes, nutmeg, cinnamon, ginger, and cloves.

Per Serving

calories: 27 | fat: 2g | protein: 1g | carbs: 4g | sugars: 1g | fiber: 2g | sodium: 4mg

Pepper Sauce

Prep time: 10 minutes | Cook time: 20 minutes | Makes 4 cups

2 red hot fresh chiles, seeded
2 dried chiles
½ small yellow onion, roughly chopped
2 garlic cloves, peeled
2 cups water
2 cups white vinegar

1. In a medium saucepan, combine the fresh and dried chiles, onion, garlic, and water. Bring to a simmer and cook for 20 minutes, or until tender. Transfer to a food processor or blender.
2. Add the vinegar and blend until smooth.

Per Serving

calories: 2 | fat: 0g | protein: 0g | carbs: 0g | sugars: 0g | fiber: 0g | sodium: 1mg

Oregano Tomato Marinara

Prep time: 5 minutes | Cook time: 15 minutes | Serves 8

1 (28-ounce / 794-g) can whole tomatoes
2 tablespoons extra-virgin olive oil
4 garlic cloves, minced
½ teaspoon salt
¼ teaspoon dried oregano

1. Discard about half of the liquid from the can of tomatoes, and transfer the tomatoes and remaining liquid to a large bowl. Use clean hands or a large spoon to break the tomatoes apart.
2. In a large skillet, heat the olive oil over medium heat. Add the garlic and salt, and cook until the garlic just begins to sizzle, without letting it brown.
3. Add the tomatoes and their liquid to the skillet.
4. Simmer the sauce for about 15 minutes until the oil begins to separate and become dark orange and the sauce thickens. Add the oregano, stir, and remove from the heat.
5. After the marinara has cooled to room temperature, store in glass containers in the refrigerator for up to 3 or 4 days, or in zip-top freezer bags for up to 4 months.

Per Serving

calories: 48 | fat: 4g | protein: 1g | carbs: 4g | sugars: 2g | fiber: 1g | sodium: 145mg

Blackened Rub

Prep time: 10 minutes | Cook time: 0 minutes | Makes about ½ cup

2 tablespoons smoked paprika
1 tablespoon sweet paprika
2 tablespoons onion powder
2 tablespoons garlic powder

1 teaspoon freshly ground black pepper
¼ teaspoon celery seeds
1 teaspoon dried dill
½ teaspoon ground mustard

1. In an airtight container, mix the smoked paprika, sweet paprika, onion powder, garlic powder, pepper, celery seeds, dill, and mustard.

Per Serving

calories: 23 | fat: 1g | protein: 1g | carbs: 5g | sugars: 1g | fiber: 1g | sodium: 3mg

Barbecue Sauce

Prep time: 5 minutes | Cook time: 15 minutes | Makes about 3 cups

1¼ cup tomato purée
1½ cup white vinegar
1 tablespoon yellow mustard
1 teaspoon mustard seeds
1 teaspoon ground turmeric
1 teaspoon sweet paprika

1 teaspoon garlic powder
1 teaspoon celery seeds
½ teaspoon cayenne pepper
½ teaspoon onion powder
½ teaspoon freshly ground black pepper

1. In a medium pot, combine the tomato purée, vinegar, mustard, mustard seeds, turmeric, paprika, garlic powder, celery seeds, cayenne, onion powder, and black pepper. Simmer over low heat for 15 minutes, or until the flavors come together.
2. Remove the sauce from the heat, and let cool for 5 minutes. Transfer to a blender, and purée until smooth.

Per Serving

calories: 7 | fat: 0g | protein: 0g | carbs: 1g | sugars: 1g | fiber: 0g | sodium: 12mg

Lime Tomato Salsa

Prep time: 10 minutes | Cook time: 0 minutes | Serves 6

2 or 3 medium, ripe tomatoes, diced
½ red onion, minced
1 serrano pepper, seeded and minced

Juice of 1 lime
¼ cup minced fresh cilantro
¼ teaspoon salt

1. In a small bowl, combine the tomatoes, onion, serrano pepper, lime juice, cilantro, and salt, and mix well. Taste and season with additional salt as needed.
2. Serve immediately, or transfer to an airtight container and refrigerate for up to 3 days.

Per Serving

calories: 18 | fat: 0g | protein: 1g | carbs: 4g | sugars: 1g | fiber: 1g | sodium: 84mg

Caramelized Onion Dip with Greek Yogurt

Prep time: 10 minutes | Cook time: 45 minutes | Serves 8

2 tablespoons extra-virgin olive oil
3 cups chopped onions
1 garlic clove, minced

2 cups plain nonfat Greek yogurt
1 teaspoon salt
Freshly ground black pepper, to taste

1. In a large pot, heat the olive oil over medium heat until shimmering. Add the onions, and stir well to coat. Reduce heat to low, cover, and cook for 45 minutes, stirring every the 5 to 10 minutes, until well-browned and caramelized. Add the garlic and stir until just fragrant.
2. Remove from the heat and let cool for 10 minutes.
3. In a mixing bowl, combine the onions, yogurt, salt, and pepper.

Per Serving

calories: 83 | fat: 4g | protein: 6g | carbs: 7g | sugars: 5g | fiber: 1g | sodium: 264mg

Garam Masala

Prep time: 5 minutes | Cook time: 0 minutes | Makes ⅓ cup

2 tablespoons ground cumin
1 tablespoon freshly ground black pepper
1 tablespoon ground cardamom
1 tablespoon ground coriander
2 teaspoons ground cinnamon
1 teaspoon ground nutmeg
1 teaspoon ground cloves
⅛ teaspoon cayenne pepper (optional)

1. In an old spice jar or small bowl, combine the cumin, black pepper, cardamom, coriander, cinnamon, nutmeg, cloves, and cayenne (if using). Mix well and store, covered and in a cool, dry location, for up to 6 months.

Per Serving (1½ tablespoons)
calories: 32 | fat: 1g | protein: 1g | carbs: 6g | sugars: 0g | fiber: 3g | sodium: 7mg

Toasted Nuts

Prep time: 1 minute | Cook time: 5 to 10 minutes | Makes ½ cup

½ cup nuts

1. Heat a dry nonstick pan over medium-high heat.
2. Place the nuts in the pan and toss or stir frequently for 2 to 5 minutes, until they are toasted and fragrant.
3. Remove from the heat and let cool.

Per Serving (1 tablespoon)
calories: 40 | fat: 3g | protein: 1g | carbs: 2g | sugars: 0g | fiber: 1g | sodium: 0mg

Low-Sodium Salsa

Prep time: 10 minutes | Cook time: 0 minutes | Makes 1 cup

8 ounces (227 g) cocktail tomatoes, quartered
2 scallions, white and light green parts only, chopped
1 jalapeño chile, seeded and chopped
2 tablespoons chopped fresh cilantro
1 tablespoon freshly squeezed lime juice

1. In a food processor, combine the tomatoes, scallions, jalapeño, cilantro, and lime juice. Pulse until the salsa is the consistency you like. If you don't have a food processor, finely chop the tomatoes, scallions, and jalapeño, then mix with the cilantro and lime juice.
2. Store, covered, in the refrigerator for up to 3 days.

Per Serving (2 tablespoons)
calories: 7 | fat: 0g | protein: 0g | carbs: 2g | sugars: 1g | fiber: 1g | sodium: 2mg

Pickled Garlic Vegetables

Prep time: 10 minutes | Cook time: 0 minutes | Makes 4 (12- to 16-ounce / 340- to 454-g) jars pickles

1 tablespoon whole allspice
1 teaspoon black peppercorns
1 tablespoon whole mustard seeds
1 teaspoon celery seeds
4 garlic cloves, smashed
7 to 10 whole okra
1 sweet onion, quartered
1 cup green beans
3 Kirby cucumbers, cut into ½-inch-thick rounds
4 cups vinegar
4 cups boiling water

1. In a small bowl, to make the dry mixture, combine the allspice, peppercorns, mustard seeds, and celery seeds.
2. Into each of four (12- to 16-ounce / 340- to 454-g) heat-proof jars, add 1 teaspoon of the dry mixture.
3. Add 1 garlic clove to each jar.
4. Fill one jar with okra, one with onion, one with green beans, and the last with cucumbers.
5. In a large bowl, mix the vinegar and boiling water.
6. Fill each jar with the vinegar and water mixture up to three-quarters full. Cover and let stand for 30 minutes, or until room temperature, then refrigerate for 24 hours. Store refrigerated for up to 2 months.

Per Serving
calories: 137 | fat: 1g | protein: 4g | carbs: 21g | sugars: 7g | fiber: 4g | sodium: 25mg

Miso-Ginger Dressing

Prep time: 10 minutes | Cook time: 0 minutes | Serves 4

1 tablespoon unseasoned rice vinegar
1 tablespoon red or white miso
1 teaspoon grated fresh ginger
1 garlic clove, minced
3 tablespoons extra-virgin olive oil

1. In a small bowl, combine the vinegar and miso into a paste. Add the ginger and garlic, and mix well. While whisking, drizzle in the olive oil.
2. Store in the refrigerator in an airtight container for up to 1 week.

Per Serving

calories: 99 | fat: 10g | protein: 1g | carbs: 1g | sugars: 0g | fiber: 0g | sodium: 169mg

Easy Italian Dressing

Prep time: 5 minutes | Cook time: 0 minutes | Serves 12

¼ cup red wine vinegar
½ cup extra-virgin olive oil
¼ teaspoon salt
¼ teaspoon freshly
ground black pepper
1 teaspoon dried Italian seasoning
1 teaspoon Dijon mustard
1 garlic clove, minced

1. In a small jar, combine the vinegar, olive oil, salt, pepper, Italian seasoning, mustard, and garlic. Close with a tight-fitting lid and shake vigorously for 1 minute.
2. Refrigerate for up to 1 week.

Per Serving

calories: 81 | fat: 9g | protein: 0g | carbs: 0g | sugars: 0g | fiber: 0g | sodium: 52mg

Vegetable Broth

Prep time: 10 minutes | Cook time: 15 minutes | Makes 8 cups

2 or 3 (4-inch) rosemary sprigs
2 or 3 (4-inch) thyme sprigs
2 or 3 (4-inch) parsley sprigs
1 large onion (unpeeled), root end trimmed, quartered
2 large carrots (unpeeled), washed,
ends trimmed, and each cut into 4 pieces
2 celery stalks (including leaves), ends trimmed and each cut into 4 pieces
4 garlic cloves, peeled and left whole
2 bay leaves
½ teaspoon peppercorns

1. Using kitchen twine, tie together the rosemary, thyme, and parsley. (If you don't have twine, don't worry about it. Tying the herbs together just makes it easier to discard them later.)
2. In the electric pressure cooker, combine the onion, carrots, celery, garlic, bay leaves, and peppercorns. Drop the herb bundle on top, then pour in 6 cups of water.
3. Close and lock the lid of the pressure cooker. Set the valve to sealing.
4. Cook on high pressure for 15 minutes.
5. When the cooking is complete, hit Cancel. Allow the pressure to release naturally for 15 minutes, then quick release any remaining pressure.
6. Once the pin drops, unlock and remove the lid.
7. Cool the broth to room temperature, then strain it through a fine-mesh strainer lined with cheesecloth. Discard the solids.
8. Transfer to storage containers and refrigerate for 3 to 4 days or freeze for up to 1 year.

Per Serving (1 cup)

calories: 12 | fat: 0g | protein: 0g | carbs: 3g | sugars: 1g | fiber: 1g | sodium: 17mg

Infused Oil and Vinegar

Prep time: 15 minutes | Cook time: 5 minutes | Makes 2 quarts

Infused Oil:

1 quart extra-virgin olive oil	1 jalapeño pepper, halved lengthwise
3 fresh thyme sprigs	6 garlic cloves, smashed
3 fresh rosemary sprigs	

Infused Vinegar:

3 fresh thyme sprigs	6 garlic cloves, smashed
3 fresh rosemary sprigs	1 quart white balsamic vinegar
1 jalapeño pepper, halved lengthwise	

Make the Infused Oil

1. In a medium saucepan, combine the oil, thyme, rosemary, jalapeño, and garlic and cook, stirring, over medium-low heat, for 3 to 5 minutes. Take care not to burn the herbs.
2. Remove the pan from the heat, and let the oil cool completely.
3. Once cooled, transfer to an airtight container and store in the refrigerator, where it will keep for up to 1 month.

Make the Infused Vinegar

1. In a large mason jar, combine the thyme, rosemary, jalapeño, and garlic.
2. Fill the jar three-quarters full with vinegar. Cover and refrigerate for 24 hours. The vinegar will be ready to use but will continue infusing. The flavor will deepen over time. Store refrigerated for up to 2 months.

Per Serving (olive oil)
calories: 113 | fat: 13g | protein: 0g | carbs: 0g | sugars: 0g | fiber: 0g | sodium: 0mg

Per Serving (vinegar)
calories: 6 | fat: 0g | protein: 0g | carbs: 0g | sugars: 0g | fiber: 0g | sodium: 0mg

Chicken Bone Broth

Prep time: 11 minutes | Cook time: 2 hours | Makes 8 cups

2 or 3 (4-inch) rosemary sprigs	ends trimmed, and each cut into 4 pieces
2 or 3 (4-inch) thyme sprigs	2 celery stalks (including leaves), ends trimmed and each cut into 4 pieces
2 or 3 (4-inch) parsley sprigs	2 bay leaves
Bones from a 3- to 4-pound (1.4- to 1.8-kg) chicken	⅛ teaspoon black peppercorns
1 large onion (unpeeled), root end trimmed, quartered	1 teaspoon kosher salt (optional)
2 large carrots (unpeeled), washed,	1 tablespoon apple cider vinegar

1. Using kitchen twine, tie together the rosemary, thyme, and parsley. (If you don't have any twine, don't worry about it. Tying the herbs together just makes it easier to discard them later.)
2. In the electric pressure cooker, combine the bones, onion, carrots, celery, bay leaves, peppercorns, and salt (if using). Drop the herb bundle on top, then add the vinegar and 8 cups of water.
3. Close and lock the lid of the pressure cooker. Set the valve to sealing.
4. Cook on high pressure for 2 hours.
5. When the cooking is complete, hit Cancel. Allow the pressure to release naturally for 20 minutes, then quick release any remaining pressure.
6. Once the pin drops, unlock and remove the lid.
7. Cool the broth to room temperature, then strain it through a fine-mesh strainer lined with cheesecloth. Discard the solids.
8. Transfer to storage containers and refrigerate for 3 to 4 days, or freeze for up to 1 year.

Per Serving (1 cup)
calories: 40 | fat: 1g | protein: 6g | carbs: 3g | sugars: 0g | fiber: 1g | sodium: 20mg

Appendix 1: Measurement Conversion Chart

VOLUME EQUIVALENTS(DRY)

US STANDARD	METRIC (APPROXIMATE)
1/8 teaspoon	0.5 mL
1/4 teaspoon	1 mL
1/2 teaspoon	2 mL
3/4 teaspoon	4 mL
1 teaspoon	5 mL
1 tablespoon	15 mL
1/4 cup	59 mL
1/2 cup	118 mL
3/4 cup	177 mL
1 cup	235 mL
2 cups	475 mL
3 cups	700 mL
4 cups	1 L

WEIGHT EQUIVALENTS

US STANDARD	METRIC (APPROXIMATE)
1 ounce	28 g
2 ounces	57 g
5 ounces	142 g
10 ounces	284 g
15 ounces	425 g
16 ounces (1 pound)	455 g
1.5 pounds	680 g
2 pounds	907 g

VOLUME EQUIVALENTS(LIQUID)

US STANDARD	US STANDARD (OUNCES)	METRIC (APPROXIMATE)
2 tablespoons	1 fl.oz.	30 mL
1/4 cup	2 fl.oz.	60 mL
1/2 cup	4 fl.oz.	120 mL
1 cup	8 fl.oz.	240 mL
1 1/2 cup	12 fl.oz.	355 mL
2 cups or 1 pint	16 fl.oz.	475 mL
4 cups or 1 quart	32 fl.oz.	1 L
1 gallon	128 fl.oz.	4 L

TEMPERATURES EQUIVALENTS

FAHRENHEIT(F)	CELSIUS(C) (APPROXIMATE)
225 °F	107 °C
250 °F	120 °C
275 °F	135 °C
300 °F	150 °C
325 °F	160 °C
350 °F	180 °C
375 °F	190 °C
400 °F	205 °C
425 °F	220 °C
450 °F	235 °C
475 °F	245 °C
500 °F	260 °C

Appendix 2: The Dirty Dozen and Clean Fifteen

The Environmental Working Group (EWG) is a nonprofit, nonpartisan organization dedicated to protecting human health and the environment Its mission is to empower people to live healthier lives in a healthier environment. This organization publishes an annual list of the twelve kinds of produce, in sequence, that have the highest amount of pesticide residue-the Dirty Dozen-as well as a list of the fifteen kinds ofproduce that have the least amount of pesticide residue-the Clean Fifteen.

THE DIRTY DOZEN	THE CLEAN FIFTEEN
• The 2016 Dirty Dozen includes the following produce. These are considered among the year's most important produce to buy organic:	• The least critical to buy organically are the Clean Fifteen list. The following are on the 2016 list:

THE DIRTY DOZEN

Strawberries	Spinach
Apples	Tomatoes
Nectarines	Bell peppers
Peaches	Cherry tomatoes
Celery	Cucumbers
Grapes	Kale/collard greens
Cherries	Hot peppers

• *The Dirty Dozen list contains two additional itemskale/collard greens and hot peppers-because they tend to contain trace levels of highly hazardous pesticides.*

THE CLEAN FIFTEEN

Avocados	Papayas
Corn	Kiw
Pineapples	Eggplant
Cabbage	Honeydew
Sweet peas	Grapefruit
Onions	Cantaloupe
Asparagus	Cauliflower
Mangos	

• *Some of the sweet corn sold in the United States are made from genetically engineered (GE) seedstock. Buy organic varieties of these crops to avoid GE produce.*

Appendix 3: Recipe Index